O9-BTM-489

HURON COUNTY LIBRARY
3 6492 00516003 8

RUN OVER

Douglas Bell

RUN OVER

A boy,

his mother,

and an accident

Random House Canada

 Published in 2001 by Random House Canada, a division of Random House of Canada Limited.

Canadian Cataloguing in Publication Data

Bell, Douglas, 1959-
Run over: a boy, his mother and an accident

ISBN 0-679-31024-X

1. Bell, Douglas, 1959- - Health.
2. Traffic accident victims – Canada – Biography.
I. Title.

RD966.B45 2001 362.1'971028'0092 C00-932460-7

Pages 223-224 constitutes a continuation of this copyright page.

Jacket design: Carmen Dunjko
Text design: Gordon Robertson Design

www.randomhouse.ca

Printed and bound in the United States of America

10 9 8 7 6 5 4 3 2 1

For my mum,
Cicely Barlow Bell,
who died October 10, 1998

The world keeps turning round and round
and leaves me hanging in the air.
My heart keeps turning upside down
and you're still standing there.

— STEVE EARLE

CONTENTS

STATEMENT OF PURPOSE

Like Samuel Beckett the survivor expresses himself *en désespoir de cause*, because there is no other way.

— ELIE WIESEL

Illness is a remedy against death, because it prepares us for death, creating an apprenticeship whose first step is self pity. Illness supports man in the great attempt to shirk the fact that he will surely die.

— ALBERT CAMUS

WHEN I THINK OF IT NOW, I think of my mother receiving the news from a uniformed cop standing at the front door of our house describing how her only child has just been crushed under the wheels of a truck. At first she's looking at the cop thinking, "Oh, crikey, he's *rawther* a large creature." And then she realizes the severity of the situation and hurries away from the door back into the house to call my father. As she goes, she's probably biting down hard on her lower lip because that's what she always does when she's angry or nervous or both.

And I remember, many years later, as she lay dying of cancer, asking her if she could recall that exact moment, and she looked at me squarely, her prominent jaw set, and said, "Oh God, Douglas, I don't know, I'd rather not remember it at all. I'd just as soon not." And I thought I might prod her a bit in the fashion of my trade, but there was something in her eyes that stopped me, a glimmer of exhaustion.

And I could see that she really didn't *want* to remember her only son that way, now, at the other end of her life, she would really rather not. And that it fell to me to make sense of things, my accident, her death and dying, to stand up and be a writer, because in the end I will be judged and not her. So that's what I'm doing. That's my statement of purpose.

ACKNOWLEDGEMENTS

THE TROUBLE WITH WRITING a book that pivots on a single (and signal) event in one's life is that some busybody's going to ask, "Okay, but what about before and what about the *rest* of your life?" It's an inconvenient though inevitable query.

In my case everything seems to turn on June 10, 1974, the day I was run over by a truck at the northeast corner of Dupont Avenue and Spadina Road in midtown Toronto. It is my life's equivalent of the big bang. Though I had a life before that moment, it seems pale and inconsequential compared with the events that followed.

Of course, just how "great" these events actually were I must leave to the reader to decide. Recently the American journalist Nicholas Lemann suggested that what he termed "the transmogrification of life into stock drama" had given rise to the ongoing spate of memoirs. "The docudrama and the novelistic lead are ubiquitous in journalism," he wrote. "The self-dramatizing memoir has taken over book publishing." And though this line of argument gave me pause, I found myself reassured by one thought: I had no choice. I had no choice getting run over by a truck. I had no choice but to watch my mother die of cancer while I contemplated these events. I had no choice but to write about it.

I use this phrase "no choice" advisedly. An esteemed writer with a painful personality once said to me that she had sacrificed her first marriage on the altar of her work. She said this out loud. I don't want to be taken to mean anything so melodramatic as that. All I mean is that, as a practical matter, I couldn't imagine writing at length about anything other than this event and the ripples it continues to throw off. The key word here is *write*. It's what I do for a living, so, for me at least, it's no small beer. But it is not life. It's not even close. When Lemann complains from the theoretical high ground that people who write memoir are doing so to be self-dramatizing, I think he's overshooting the mark. He's assuming there's some grand process in play to which writers wittingly or unwittingly fall victim. And for a smart journalist like Lemann that's a good thing—he's letting the light into the secret world that needs to be revealed every morning or every week or every month. My view is that the true unmediated course of things is all too confusing and convoluted to be "revealed." It is only to be wrestled with. Writing, like travelling or parenting or collecting porcelain, is just another way of holding off mortification. In a recent paean to the American novelist Frederick Exley, D.J. Taylor caught exactly the important difference I am here discussing. "For some reason," he wrote in *The Guardian*, "*look at me being a man* is always a more interesting command than *look at me being a writer*."

All of which reminds me: I am alive, which under the circumstances is a pretty good deal. And because I am alive I get a chance to acknowledge people who for whatever reason have helped me write this book. Which, let's face it, is one of the few times one can, with unencumbered sincerity, appear gracious.

First to my editor and friend Anne Collins, whose patience, generous nature and kindness have known no match in my professional life.

To the tolerant and generous souls at Random House of Canada who put up with me hanging around the office for lo those many months: especially, John Neale, Maya Mavjee, Martha Kanya-Forstner, David Kent, Pam Robertson and Debbie Gaudet. To John Fraser, who offered his good offices as master of Massey College in support of a guy who'd spent no small portion of John's editorial budget at *Saturday Night* chasing a story that never got done. His is the triumph of faith over a credit check. To Ian Brown, for suggesting I write for a living and for everything else. To Michael Ignatieff and Don Obe for cracking the bottle of champagne over this vessel. To generous colleagues Evan Solomon, Mark Kingwell, Meg Murphy, Tim Falconer, Douglas Coupland, Robert and John Colapinto, Moira Farr, Jennifer Baichwal, Andy Heintzman, Ken Finkleman, Anna Luengo, Matthew Church, Jenny Marcus, Patricia Pearson, Stephanie Miller, Patrick Graham, Don Gillmor and Ellen Vanstone. To the Stoneys of Rosturk Woods, Ireland, and also to the Sinclairs of Laguna Beach, California. To my agent, Bruce Westwood.

To Doctors Greenberg, Harrison, Ein, McCann, Cohen, Hegarty and Fleming.

To my friends John Sinclair, John Hendra, Marcus Pratt, Ivor Elrifi, Norm Farrell, Ken Alexander, Mike Guy and Stewart Young, who prove year in and year out that loyalty is its own reward.

To my very smart wife and friend, Jean Gilchrist, and my children Anne and Charlotte (who, aged six, offered unsolicited an alternate title for this book—*Boom, Boom Crash: Nobody's Going to Buy This Book*). To my dad, Norman Bell; to the late Jim Cormier and all other absent friends. Your devotion flatters me and your affection sustains me.

RUN

PART 1

OVER

BIRTH

IT WAS A STORY he asked her for all the time when he was small. *Tell me about when I was born* he asked *tell me again please*.

"You came out early," she said. "Several weeks early." The doctors didn't believe she was in labour at first. They told her she was hysterical, that she needed to go home and rest up for the real thing. They gave her some Valium to help move her along. But he arrived anyway. He came out floppy like a fresh fish arriving on ice to market. And he spent his first few days on this earth in an incubator, small and fragile, but he survived, not like the others, and soon became his mother's little angel.

LATER

To the happy and the well born and the rich he had this to say—that for all their affection their comforts and their privileges they would not be spared the pangs of anger and lust and the agonies of death. He only meant for them to be prepared for the blow when the blow fell. But was it not possible to accept this truth without having him dance a jig in your living room?

— JOHN CHEEVER, "The Scarlet Moving Van"

MINE WAS A COMFORTABLE upbringing. I use that term cautiously. I picked it up from Conrad Black's autobiography. In his case it was meant to signal that his is a riches-to-greater-riches story. Mine has nothing to do with getting from or to anywhere. It's hardly even a story, really, more like a boxful of family photographs spilled out on the carpet. I make the story up as each image reminds me of this or that.

Growing up, we were wealthy. Not as wealthy as Conrad Black, mind you, but "comfortable." Lately, I've discovered how we got to be that way. I've started to wrestle with the fact that my forebears were more than just comfortable; they were filthy rich. A book titled *The Estates of Old Toronto* clued me in. The book describes seventy-one of

Toronto's great estates. Its contents fall somewhere between nostalgia and history, tending to a treacly treatment of wealth gone by. "Up the winding drive, a rustle of long skirts, and the muffled crunch of gravel underfoot heralds arrival at the country estate . . ." Page 142 reveals a photograph of Sunnybrook Farm, an enormous country house that sat on the property where Toronto's Sunnybrook Hospital sits today.

"Sunnybrook House was a large rambling affair with several wings. Inside, oak panelling, an open gallery, beamed ceilings and hunting trophies created the flavour of an English country manor . . . Alice and Joseph Kilgour had no children, so when he died his widow donated Sunnybrook Farm to the city to be used as a park. Alice transferred the 172 acres in 1928 . . . There was one stipulation attached to Mrs. Kilgour's gift: any use of the land for purposes other than a park would have to be approved by the Kilgour [heirs]."

As luck would have it, I am, on my father's side, one of those heirs.

It's an odd sensation knowing that you come from a great deal of power, privilege and money, and yet thanks to a whimsical turn in your great-great-aunt's fancy (an aunt who, despite that turn, was still known to subsequent generations as "Aunt Alice from whom all blessings flow") your potential station was reduced in a moment from hilariously rich to "comfortable." (When I say "odd sensation," I mean to say that inherited wealth reminds you life is fundamentally inequitable, and yet no matter how advantaged one's situation one always imagines it might be better.)

I can't remember my father mentioning this bequest in any other light than the obligations bearing on the heirs—except once. (My father's obligations were considerable and he dealt with them brilliantly. He rose to be chairman of Sunnybrook Hospital, and in recognition of his service to the hospital and his exemplary war record he received an honorary doctorate from his alma mater, Trinity College.) I was in my mid-thirties and we were driving along the south end of the property. I asked dad how far it extended. Gazing into the middle distance, he wondered aloud, "Can you imagine if Alice had just hung on to some of it? My God. We'd none of us have had to work a day." It was all he could do to shake his head, clear his mind and keep the car on the road as we continued along Eglinton Avenue West before turning north at the western end of the property.

Exploring the depths of my father's conservatism could easily merit a book of its own. He was and is a cautious realist, with the emphasis on caution. His experience in wartime taught him to prepare for the worst. Hence, throughout the sixties and seventies, ours was a two-bomb-shelter family—one in Toronto and one at the cottage. These came complete with self-sustaining air and water filtration systems. There were several hundred tins of canned food. I seem to remember a lot of brown beans. This stimulated my imagination as to just how truly dreadful life would be after a nuclear holocaust. The beds swung down from the wall on chains. And of course there was oodles of rat poison. My father was never shy of expressing himself on the horrors that awaited anyone who dared to venture uninvited to share our facilities in the aftermath of an A-bomb. It always seemed to involve my standing at the entryway, pistol at the ready to fire on the rascals, those laggards who hadn't the wit to "think ahead."

Mum had been born to a similar sort of privilege, in somewhat different circumstances. She grew up in various parts of Upper and Lower Canada. Her father was an up-and-coming engineer (he would later become chairman and CEO of the paper giant Abitibi-Price) living and working in places like Iroquois Falls, Sarnia, Thorold, St. Catharines and Quebec City. (It was in the latter locale that mum, on an extremely cold morning in a curious frame of mind, stuck out her tongue and attached it to the steel letter box affixed to the side of her house. Warm water helped resolve the situation, but not before mum had left a considerable portion of her tongue on the box. She told me this story early in life, and though I've often been tempted, I have continued to honour the cautionary aspect of that tale.)

Mum was home-schooled by a governess till the age of twelve, then eventually sent off to Havergal College for Girls in Toronto before going on to join the pearl-and-sweater set at McGill University. Sheila Bourke, who was a classmate of my mum's and went on to become a librarian at McGill, remembered mum in a letter following her death: "My mother used to lecture your mother when she would arrive at our house in the depths of winter wearing high-heeled shoes to walk through the snow. Of course we both smoked in those days, your mother smoking American cigarettes, and I can still see the way she opened the package, with her pretty hands, peeling back the shiny paper in a small square and tapping out a cigarette." My grandparents, who in the late forties settled once and for all in Toronto, lived in a massive house perched on a cliff in Toronto's slightly eccentric though still wealthy enclave, Wychwood Park.

By any reasonable standard, comfortable still meant rich. During my first year at St. George's College, a private boys' school in midtown Toronto, my parents went away for a couple of weeks. I was left in the care of a nanny who didn't, or wouldn't, drive. Every day a large black limousine complete with uniformed driver from a company called Cullitons turned up at the house to deliver me to school. (For some time afterwards I referred to limousines in general as Cullitons.) This rapidly turned into a fiasco when several schoolmates saw me emerging, bright red Thermos lunch box in hand. Word got round and one teacher in particular, David McMaster, himself a product of inherited wealth, started giving me a hard time. One day while I was kicking a soccer ball about with some other boys, he announced to a group of my chums that "his lordship's train has arrived." This had a somewhat alienating effect on my friends.

In the following days I begged the driver to let me off farther and farther away from the school, to the point where I was actually late as a result. Turning up at the door of the registrar (a big man with slick silver and black hair and a tart tongue, known to all as "the Bear"), I first demonstrated my Wile E. Coyote–like genius for excuse making. The exchange went something like this:

Me: Sir, the, uh, car I was in was in an, ummmm, accident and I had to, ahhhh ahhhh, walk the rest of the way.

The Bear: First of all, that's not a car, it's a limousine. Second, if I call Cullitons, they better confirm your story.

Me: Okay, okay, okay. Look, uh, accident's a strong word, perhaps too strong... Still, there was a lot of traffic....

A couple of weeks later McMaster confronted my mother at a parent–teacher meeting and suggested that sending her child to school in a limousine could put distance between Doug and his peers. Mother's initial response, I remember, was something in the range of "fuck off," later amended to, "I suppose it makes some sense. Still, the temerity of that pipsqueak." Soon enough I was taking advice from mother on the ins and outs of public transportation, a service she knew little about. I remember standing forlornly on the platform at the corner of Bathurst and St. Clair waiting for a streetcar with a sign that read, specifically, "St. Clair-Eglinton." I could have jumped on any streetcar that came by, but mum had taken literal note of some instruction or other and persuaded me that if I were to take any streetcar other than one marked "St. Clair-Eglinton," I would fall into the hands of Turkish highway bandits, or worse. I waited a long time, watching white snowflakes blur together into a golden mass as they fell under the gaze of a yellow signal lamp at the end of the platform.

Several years later, Grade 11 maybe, I took a course portentously titled "Man in Society" and given by that same McMaster. There was a session devoted to class and its role in determining one's place in the greater scheme of things. At a boys' private school in downtown Toronto the students with one exception selected themselves as middle class. The exception was me. I selected the upper class as my natural domain. Seeking company for my lonely status, I argued that, based on percentages, my classmates' families had to be in the upper tier of income earners and were therefore upper class. Neither my confreres nor McMaster would have any of it. I realize now that it was my mother's disdain for the middle class that drove me to object. Whenever she uttered those words—*middle class*—she did so with the same inflection she might have used to describe dog crap on her shoe. And though I suppose my mother was as capable as anyone of her class and disposition of harbouring the sort of ill will that this sentiment implies, the better angels of her nature gave voice to pure liberalism. It was the kind of liberalism that objects to classification, period. I sometimes wonder whether mum wasn't a closet anarchist the way her shoulders hunched with rage every time she heard politicians of any stripe talk about "ordinary" Canadians.

As a boy of seven or eight I once asked my mother about my forebears. "Did they have money?"

Not too many years later that same question might have elicited a curt glance followed by, "Douglas, don't be so crass." However, I was just young enough to merit a considered response.

"Well," my mother said, using the particularly contrived British diction she reserved for acute remarks, "it's not that they were rich so much as they were educated." Educated, in this sense, means discerning—knowing, that is to say, the differences between us and them; *us* meaning people who "know how to behave" and *them* meaning those who don't. My parents (my mother especially) were snobs, but they were discerning snobs, and that makes a difference. Or at least enough of a difference that, despite my anarchic leanings, I still loved them quite a lot.

If I accused my mother of being a snob, she would laugh merrily and say, "Of *course* I'm a snob." Unspoken was that my use of the word *snob* as a term of derision was to her mind trivial, as in "Of course I'm a snob. Some people are simply better bred than others. Anyone knows that."

Today I understand that what mum really meant was that self-interest dictates that certain presumptions regarding a person's character and ability, based on appearances, are necessary in order to discern that person's place in the scheme of things. Nothing wrong with that. (Of course there *is* something wrong with that, but I still haven't managed to shake that particular regulation of my upbringing.) What my mother and I disagreed about were the criteria for those presumptions, and more importantly, the proviso that one never, ever, discuss them. It's the Catch-22 of my inherited world view: if you have to ask, you clearly don't deserve to know.

This was a leitmotif for my mother on subjects that distinguished *us* from *them*. The most obvious example was her unwillingness to countenance anything she deemed "common." Mum's list of the common would rival the Domesday Book. To wit: commenting generally on how you "feel" about things was taboo. A declarative statement like "I'm not feeling very good about life at the moment" would result in her snappish response, "And who, pray tell, does?" Beyond the states of mind deemed "not on" were a welter of pronunciations and expressions that situated one instantly in my mother's eyes. Take the pronunciation of Montreal. If you drag out the vowels and pronounce it *Maaaawwn-treaaaawwwwwl* with the emphasis on *awwwwwl*, you're one of us; if you pronounce it *Munt-tree-all* like every other English-speaking person in the country (clipped; *Munt* rhymes with *bunt*)—well, you're one of them. Similarly:

curtains *us*	drapes *them*
sofa *us*	couch *them*
house *us*	home *them*
de-fence *us*	dee-fence *them*
not a bit *us*	you're welcome *them*
sorry *us*	I beg your pardon *them*

I could go on.

Another way of thinking about this is captured by one of my mother's favourite phrases, trotted out whenever she wanted to be emphatic or conclusive on just about any subject: *comme il faut*. Literally, it means "how it must be." That's the thing about class as a way of discerning how to live in the world: all the questions are answered before they're asked. Things aren't just the way they are, they are how they *must* be. The unexamined life isn't worth examining.

Comme il faut was manifested in where my mother went to buy things or to get things done. It seemed there was always somewhere that was just exactly the right place to go to get whatever it was one wanted. My mother patronized *the* (pronounced *theeee*) hairdresser, Gerald; *the* dressmaker, Zoe; *the* food shop, Chez Charbon; *the* grocer, Bilton's; *the* hardware store, Irwin's; *the* French tutor, Madame Soutzo (a genuine Romanian princess); *the* children's shoe shop, The Three Little Pigs; *the* boys' clothing store, Beattie's; *the* boys' summer camp, Hurontario; *the* auction house, Waddington's; *the* jewellery shop, Secrett's. *The* certainty that everything with which she had contact was far and away the best (and more than the best, the *only*) had a weird effect on me as a kid. Whenever I came across anyone, anywhere, doing anything other than *comme il faut*, I was immediately suspicious. This extended to the brand of cigarettes or beer that other kids' parents smoked and drank.

"What? You don't smoke Craven 'A'? How . . . odd."

"That's not Molson's Export you're drinking, is it? Strange."

My mother's prejudices weren't limited to fine distinctions of lexicon, pronunciation and consumerism. One of my favourite Monty Python skits revolves around a parody of BBC documentaries and features the bad doings of the infamous criminal siblings Doug and Dinsdale Piranha. The Piranhas are extremely violent to the point where one victim testifies to having had his head nailed to the floor. "Why?" asks the guileless interviewer. "Well, he had to, didn't he?" replies the addled victim. "I mean, be fair. There was nothing else he could do. I mean, I had transgressed the unwritten law . . . He was a cruel man . . . but fair." This, I've always thought, was a neat analogy for my mother's views on the wider world of propriety.

For instance, Patricia, my half-sister from my father's first marriage, had difficulties in her personal life and was the constant subject of my mother's disapprobation. The following diatribe was delivered hard on the heels of Patricia's decision to live with a newly acquired boyfriend. She'd met the boyfriend while taking instruction from him in figure skating. "They're going to live together, and for God's sake, he's the *skating instructor* at the *Granite* Club." Parsing this declaration of high snobbery requires the legerdemain of an Irish historian. That they were going to live together outside marriage was bad. That he was a skating instructor was worse. But that he was a skating instructor at the *Granite Club*—well, that was worst of all. First off, Patricia was a member of that club, and getting involved with one of the staff was not on. Compounding the sin was that Patricia was a member of that club at all. The Granite was considered, by my mother at least, to be second-tier, full of parvenus and other dubious sorts (insurance agents, dentists, tradespeople, etc.). The thought that people of that ilk might look down their noses at Patricia and, by extension, at my mother was definitely not on.

Here's how I found out I even *had* a half-sister. Until I was eight years old I assumed my sister, whom I called my sister, was, well, my sister. Then my sister went to university. A while after that my parents got angry, very angry, all the time. I had no idea what this was about, except I knew they were unhappy with Patricia but were taking it out on me. My name changed from Douglas to "go to your room." This went on for months, it seemed. One day the kitchen phone rang. I couldn't reach it comfortably from the floor, so I clambered up on a chair (one of those moulded one-piece Swedish modern jobs) and took the call. The voice on the other end asked to speak to her daughter Patricia. "That's funny," I said, "because I have a sister, but she couldn't be *your* daughter because she's *my* sister." There was a long pause. The voice said, betraying a certain impatience, "My name is Sally Hay and I'd like to speak to *my* daughter Patricia." I started to repeat that, though she might well have a daughter named Patricia, it couldn't be the same Patricia since my sister's mother—that is to say *my* mother—was just down the hall. Would you like to speak to her?

In the midst of this my dad opened the swinging kitchen door from the dining room. He seemed to get the situation all in one go. Then, the way I tell it, it was as though my dad were the elastic man from the Marvel comic strip *The Fantastic Four*. He seemed to stretch his arms across the kitchen, grab me and the phone all in one motion and, while muttering darkly into the receiver, gently place me in the dog cage beneath the chair. The cage door closed, the lock snapped shut and, while he went on talking, I wrapped my hands around the bars and peered up at my father's intent expression. It was only years later that I learned in an explicit sense that my father had been married before.

None of this could be discussed. If I so much as suggested that none of it really mattered relative to my half-sister's happiness, my mother would look into the middle distance, suck in her cheeks and through violently clenched teeth announce, "I haven't the *faintest* idea what you're talking about," the clear implication being "and neither do you."

And I didn't really. The subtleties of my mother's social calculus were a mystery, thanks to the prime directive. To this day I continue to see it at best through a glass, darkly.

There was always with my mother the sense that we had been exiled from the metropolis. The all-seeing, all-powerful shamans, the people who really knew how to behave, lived across an ocean. My mother held in awestruck veneration a series of tony friends in Britain whom she had carefully cultivated through the course of her life. There were family connections stretching back at least a generation previous: my maternal grandmother had served tea to the Queen on one of Her Majesty's early jaunts across Canada. The British connections had names like Gladstone (great-grandson of the prime minister), Pelham (Eton man), Wrong (director of the Barbican Centre) and Stormonth-Darling (a senior executive at one of Britain's most venerated financial houses and brother of the man who at one stage oversaw the Queen's investments). My mother's bookshelves were thick with biographies, autobiographies, journals and diaries by various Sitwells, Bloomsburys, royals and so on. I think of that library now as a sort of syllabus for social propriety. Whenever mum discussed a book of which she approved, there was always an underlying pedantic advisory: If you would only read this, you too might learn how to behave.

Near the end of her life mum made a fuss over a book titled *August & Rab* ("beautifully written, articulate and published by Weidenfeld and Nicolson, who do *all* the best books"—meaning books about and by royals and aristocrats). Then suddenly her tone shifted and her voice took on a brittle timbre. The book belonged to a Mrs. Betsy Mason of Oaklawn Gardens and *had* to be returned . . . *promptly*. The book, it seemed, was a kind of object lesson. If I had managed to return it *promptly*, then I suppose I would have learned the lesson inhering in it. As I couldn't bring myself to open the book for eight months after mum died, I failed to learn my mother's cryptic lesson. And when I did read it, it was a lot like any good book, so much more than anything you might possibly have expected because expecting isn't reading—or living, for that matter.

August & Rab is the memoir of Mollie Butler, a woman who married two leading figures in twentieth-century British life. August Courtauld was the quintessential British adventurer. His heroism was the sort that brooks no dispute. On an expedition to map air routes across the polar north, Courtauld relieved two mates from a base camp and volunteered to stay on the ice for five months so that his compatriots would have enough provisions for the return trip. For a moment he was among the most famous men in the world as his British colleagues raced across Greenland's frozen horizons searching him out, a single man buried in the ice. Butler writes of this period with a pitch-perfect combination of devotion and sheer admiration. Later, August dies young of MS and Mollie goes on to marry, in mid-life, Rab Butler, generally conceded to be the greatest prime minister Britain never had—too smart, too dutiful, too engaged and too amused for the brass ring, a saint in politician's clothing. In sum: two great men married to a devoted wife smart enough to write a book that captures their essential brilliance, decency and charm not only as individuals but as married men.

As I read along, I imagined this was a sort of postcard from my mother, each telling phrase and thought an emphatic description of her Arcadian ideal. I can hear her: "Such accomplished people. Here, let me read this, have you got a minute?"

> We usually went twice a term to Gatcomb, a house in Gloucestershire which had been left to Rab in the 1940s ["I've seen that house, it's heavenly," said my mother], of which he was very fond. Rab was an example of the adage, "a sense of possession turns all to gold". . . In a technological society in which material plenty is matched by spiritual starvation, [the arts] remind us of the existence of a higher order of values and of further heights to which the human spirit can be elevated . . . and then one day Rab said the most marvellous thing to me. He said, "I am very interested in the romance of marriage. If you love someone you don't notice or mind anything. It is the most wonderful institution if interpreted properly." I set this down as a testimonial to old age.

This was exactly the sort of thinking and writing my mother adored: cool, detached, yet keenly observant of how the great and the good conduct their affairs. I can see her brow wrinkling with pleasure and her saying to me, perhaps while I sat at the end of her bed, her black eyes peering intently over the edge of her half glasses, "Isn't it delicious—so civilized." And yet in the same moment as I imagine her pleasure, I see her eyes flicker somewhere between sadness, anger and disappointment. Things hadn't quite turned out that way for her, and Mollie Butler was a distant light who served to remind mum more of the harshness of the sea than the way to the shore.

My mother's life in a conventional sense was eventful and admirable. She was an established figure in the circle of clubby Anglican Toronto. Though there's a public record of her involvements and accomplishments that would choke a horse, what I remember are the totems: the sound of her old typewriter clacking in the basement as friends gathered to organize some event or other (she was co-founder of the National Ballet School Scholarship Fund); French newspapers from places like Hawkesbury and Cornwall piling up in the garage (she was a member of a government commission on minority language rights in Ontario); her railing at the dinner table against her nemesis Bob McMichael, "the man is an utter and absolute philistine" (she was chairman of the board of the McMichael Gallery).

And yet somehow mum was never quite *of* it. There was about her a wry contempt for the pretensions of Old Toronto (or OT) full of its FOOFs (Fine Old Ontario Families) and NQOSDs (Not Quite Our Sort Dear). I always suspected that her renegade streak came from a deep sense of just how arbitrary and fickle were the categories of class and position. She told me several times the story of her birth, how her mother had clambered on a train from Iroquois

Falls (where her husband was working as an engineer) and made the 500-mile trip to Montreal, "just so I might have a decent address." Still, mum knew that pretension, pomposity and self-importance were rooted in where you came from and who you knew, and whether any of it took hold sufficiently that you learned to behave. There was a saying she uttered often enough that, like a child's prayer, its meaning dissolved into its pace and rhythm: "You only," she would say, her voice sliding easily but emphatically to a thunderous conclusion, "have your good name *once*."

Layered on top of these certainties was her tremendous, charismatic energy, and she had a ton of friends on whom to bestow it. When I was a boy, she used to take me on her rounds of Christmas gift giving, dropping off prizes, as she called them, to acquaintances all over the city and beyond. I remember particularly her women friends, their names like the Latin names of flowers, rich in meaning and resonance—Cherith Howard, June Barrett, Nancy Prescott, Dorry Dunlop, Marrietta Freeman-Attwood—each of them connected in humour, grace, prejudice and endeavour to the latticework of my mother's life and mind. I remember her wrenching the wheel of her Volkswagen around, punctuating each yank with another layer of complaint at the arduousness of this task. "Next... time ... we're get... ting ... pow... werrsteer... ing. Bloo... dy Hell! What a per... for... mance." But her ardour always belied her complaint, as she willed her "sewing machine" onward to the next appointment.

All the time I was growing up, it seemed that my mother wasn't quite where she was meant to be. She wasn't so much possessed of a world view as of a *Weltschmerz* that infected everything. By her own account my mother was rarely confused. Angry yes, confused hardly. And yet even where confusion was clearly the case, mum simply translated her anxieties and discombobulation into an argot she could at least understand, if not take comfort from.

My most vivid memory of this attitude was her inadvertent revelation of what I thought at the time must have been or should have been a dark family secret. The occasion was a happy one, a dinner party with friends and some family. I was twelve or so. Mum was wearing a festive red silk gown with a plunging neckline. Somehow the Kennedy assassination came up. Mum was in a gay G and T frame of mind straight out of Cheever. "Will you ever forget? Gracious. That was an awful week." She paused and momentarily swung her attention my way. "*You*," she said emphatically, as though it were an endearment, "had pneumonia and I had a miscarriage."

That word struck me like an axe. I kept looking at my mother all the way through dinner with something like grief. I was angry because she had told other people (not even relations) about something that seemed so private. Later she came into my room while I lay in bed and asked if there was anything the matter. I was, in the manner of most preadolescents, astonished that my mother had noticed anything about me, and at first I simply denied there was anything wrong. After she gently chided me, I found myself saying, "Well, it's kind of a big thing finding out that somebody died."

And suddenly I was mourning my dead sibling, imagining an entire world that never was.

But I was young and it was all too immense, so I immediately shut it off. And then, almost as an afterthought, my mother in a breezy tone, confided that she'd had lots of miscarriages, as if it wasn't anything to worry about. With that, as she liked to say about other abrupt encounters, my mother swept off.

Now as I think of it, it's still immense. And I can't console myself with the idea that I'll eventually grow to understand its contours and implications. You see, ever since my mother died, I wonder constantly what it was that was running through her head at the end. And I wonder whether me minus several dead babies equals consolation. And then I think of her sitting at the end of my bed after the accident, while I was in the intensive care unit of the Hospital for Sick Children, another wounded baby. And when I think of it, it's like looking at the stars. First you wonder and then you dread and then you look away.

I'm sure she would think all this gazing at stars and entrails indulgent. "If," I can imagine my mother's darkest inner voice whispering to the void, "people only knew how to behave."

Ever since I can remember, I've thought of myself as both lazy and profoundly incompetent. When my mother told me that soon I would be heading off to nursery school, I felt disquieted and underwhelmed. I'd heard some distant rumour about school and it did not engage me. I remember thinking, "That sounds like a lot of work."

On that first day my mother took me by the hand and walked me down Avenue Road, past the bronze statue of Peter Pan in the park where I played happily most days, to the school a couple of blocks south of our house. There's a photo of me and mum taken that morning. I'm dressed in a pale blue double-breasted coat and pale blue rimmed cap.

It was a French immersion school, and that first morning I was introduced to a new language by way of flash cards. (Why a French school? Mum had grown up in Quebec and had wanted to be a translator.) The teacher held up a picture of an apple. "Pomme," some kid cried out. She held up a potato. "Pomme de terre," yelped another. I was struck by two thoughts: (a) How do these kids know this stuff? and (b) (more urgently) I have to go to the bathroom.

I raised my hand. The teacher ignored me as flash card after flash card was displayed bearing the likeness of various *fruits et légumes*. I strained, holding my right arm up with my left hand. Suddenly it was too late. My arm continued to strain skyward. The teacher held up a picture of an orange. "Alors?" she asked, raising an eyebrow while pushing the picture of the citrus forward.

"Can I go unh-unh?" ("Unh-unh" was the high church version of "poo.") There was a buzz around the room.

"Hokay," she said with a comical French accent, "you alwayz muzt go to zee bazzrume bevore zee clazz, hokay?" There was a long silence as I continued to look at her beseechingly. Finally she nodded and I was out the door *vite vite*, penguining along towards the *toilette*. Once inside, I reasoned that the whole ball of wax had to go in the bowl, underwear and all. While dropping it in, I made the whistling sound of a falling bomb. Then I flushed. The water rose and continued to rise, up to the edge of the bowl and over. I felt a surge of panic and thought it best to get the hell out of there, but not before I'd rescued the sopping mess and dropped it into a nearby garbage can. As I exited the scene, I could still hear the water sloshing onto the floor.

Having resumed my seat, I later witnessed an animated conversation at the door between my teacher and a colleague.

She looked flustered, jerking her eyes towards us every so often. She asked the class if anyone had left their underwear in the bathroom. I looked steadfastly at the floor and said *rien*.

My mother used to dine out on a story about how I'd come back to the house after my first day at school and announced that I would take a pass on day two, thanks. Mum thought this was hilarious.

After four years at the French school I wrote the entrance exam for Upper Canada College, the ne plus ultra of Canadian private education for boys. My father and my father's father had attended. By any usual standard this made me a fairly solid bet for a legacy spot.

I flunked so spectacularly that even the prospect of a wealthy patron who would have donated plenty of cash to help keep the wolves from the door couldn't get me in. The magnitude of my failure was there for me to see in a letter from the junior school headmaster, a guy named Dick Howard. (Imagine going through life with a name like Dick Howard.) Dad had left it out on the glass-topped bar from which he took his evening drink. I seem to remember a word like *substandard* jumping out at me and a sickening sense that I had disappointed somebody. At nine, words like substandard disperse through you as quickly as they appear. You accept as fact your failings—the argument becomes the premise—and you carry on, merrily compensating all the way.

Later I took pains to eavesdrop on mum and dad's every conversation concerning my academic progress or lack of it, crouched outside the living-room door in my pinstriped cotton pajamas as my parents, drinking gin and Scotch, discussed their failures and mine. We lived in an enormous mock Tudor duplex at the corner of Lonsdale and Avenue roads (a relative lived in the other half). The interior was designed, my mother used to say, like the *Queen Mary*. Our half of the house was in essence one long broadloomed hallway, with a tiny living room at one end (mum called it the fishbowl), then an enormous drawing room (where the orchestra no doubt would have played had we gone down), then (through a wide, square doorway) a receiving hall. At this point you had to negotiate a tight S turn; down a long, narrow hallway past the turn were the stairs to a basement dungeon (my playroom) and the bedrooms and washrooms beyond.

As a little boy of five I used to belt up and down the length of the house in a football helmet, duffle coat and kilt complete with sporran. Shortly after bedtime, between the ages of ten and thirteen, I used to sneak down that same taupe broadloom, alert to every squeak and groan and how to avoid them. I would settle beside the doorway and listen to the straight goods on friends, relatives, business partners and their wives. Though I can't remember many specifics, I do recall the sense that this was how adults really spoke. Nothing hedged, no talking down, no lessons learned—simply acute observations on the passing parade. (Booze fuelled all forms of social discourse. A letter from a friend of the family describes a typical round of evening libation: "I had an introduction to martinis with your mother and father, never having had one in life before. We spent a weekend with them at Lake Simcoe; dinner was preceded by a martini, sherry with the soup, wine during dinner, and a liqueur after dinner, and if that wasn't sufficient we played bridge and had a drink. I still remember how terrible I felt the next morning and have never looked a martini in the eye since.")

Still, there were some uncomfortable moments. My parents' discussion of the French school's failure to provide me with even rudimentary math and English skills was summarized neatly by my mother: "The French school was an unmitigated disaster, but that still leaves the question, what *are* we going to do about it?" There was an uncomfortable silence, and then my father harrumphed and stood up to make his way to bed. I scampered down the hall, slipping sideways into the bedroom in two long strides and diving under the covers. As I settled into a phony slumber (complete with deep breathing), my dad entered my room, opened the window a smidgen wider, retreated to the doorway and watched me (fake) sleep.

What are we going to do about him?

I remember the first time I felt my mother's insistent love, the tone of it, the warp and woof of it. One afternoon at the cottage (a sprawling pile set amidst several acres of hedged gardens on the south shore of Lake Simcoe, about an hour north of Toronto) I am snooping through the medicine cabinet in my mother's bathroom. I am about three or four. I discover some capsules, which I twist apart and dump into a tumbler full of water. They make a fizzing sound as the contents dissolve. I watch the whirling, bubbling pattern of the water for what seems a very long time. Eventually I dump the contents down the drain.

Next thing, I am telling mum about twisting the caps open, as though reporting the results of a scientific experiment. Suddenly her face is full of hysterical energy. "Did you swallow?" she asks, gripping my arms with her hands and shaking me. "Did you swallow? Did you? Did you swallow?" Her voice has the quality of a siren, and for some reason I picture swallows spraying out of a tree.

Now we are driving to the clinic several miles away, in Jacksons Point. As we slow to take a corner, her hand reaches instinctively across the space between to rest against my chest, keeping me pinned to the seat. As she drives she chews her lower lip and looks at me with some wild thought playing behind her brown eyes. As it happens, the doctor has a tin of powdered Keen's mustard, which he empties into a cup of water, stirs and then insists I swallow. This in turn empties my stomach of its contents. By the time this has played out, my mother is emptied of her panic, exhausted by the ferocity of her will.

Even then the intensity of my mother's protectiveness seemed crazy to me. I remember wondering what I could possibly do to placate her, to calm her rage.

That was the face of my mother's love. Fierce and angry. All the time.

One evening in grade school I walked over to the snow-covered playing fields of Upper Canada College to go sliding down a hill on a silver saucer. Then I stopped to watch a hockey practice on the school's outdoor rink. I watched and watched until the players left the ice, and then I watched as the boys re-emerged from the hut in which they'd changed, wandered back onto the ice and began to play shinny in their shiny galoshes, their navy blue and dun-coloured duffle coats flapping open and closed as they deked and dodged.

After the last of them left the ice, I started for home. But I walked slowly, intoxicated by the sheer thrill of being late, of walking in the pitch cold dark. I stopped on the road that led to the college's front gates, fifty yards from the house, and lay back on a snowbank and stared at the stars. "I'm really late," I said to myself. "I'm really *really* late."

Just then I was picked up by the scruff. It was Ethel, our West Indian housekeeper. She dragged me home, repeating all the way, "Fool chile make you mudder sick wid worry." Ethel dropped me in the hall in front of my father, wearing his worsted wool topcoat and brown fedora. "What do you think you're doing?" he asked, his face twisting with annoyance.

Bundled up in her mink stole, a diamond bracelet flashing in the light of the front-hall chandelier, my mother stood shaking, her face a mask that showed no relief at my appearance. Her mouth was a red slash of lipstick that jerked this way and that. She raced out behind dad without a word. And I wondered, why is she so angry?

When I was twelve, mum took me along with my cousin Geoff (my "twin," born the same day as me, December 12, 1959) on a trip to New York City and Washington, D.C. In New York we stayed at a private club just off Fifth Avenue, around the corner from the Pierre Hotel. The rooms were enormous, the snow-white bedding contrasting with the dark, thick-limbed Edwardian furniture.

I remember the feeling of euphoria as we walked between office towers, my head craning every which way to see the tops of things, and mum snapping off cigarette after cigarette, the smoke causing her eyelids to flutter. She was telling and showing us everything at once: the Empire State Building, the art deco interiors of the Rockefeller Center, Atlas with the world on his back, the Met, the Guggenheim, Central Park, the shop windows along Fifth Avenue. She fired out endless details and watched it bounce off our twelve-year-old skulls like hail off the roof of a cab.

One afternoon we visited the Lila Acheson Center at the Bronx Zoo, an enormous indoor sanctuary where exotic birds flew about our heads. I noted the birds and the foliage reflected in mum's glasses as she swivelled her head this way and that. "Isn't it splendid?" she asked. As we wandered, I became aware that Geoff wanted to run away. He was bored hauling his twelve-year-old self around at his aunt's beck and call, and he'd had enough. Suddenly he was off at full speed, and I was after him. And so it went, with Geoff off like a hare ahead of the hounds and me chasing him all over the zoo.

Each time I sought to drag him back, he would say something provocative to weaken my own resolve, to make me question whether I shouldn't be taking a crack at running away too.

"Let's go. We can be outta here and downtown before she knows what hit her."

"Geoff, shut up will ya. Mum's getting really mad. Please come back . . . *plleeeaaassse*."

We managed to get out the other end intact, Geoff pulling away, me hanging on to his jacket and mum hanging on to me, moving together like a racing sloop heeling as she heads into the wind. We found ourselves out on Fordham Road, near the Bronx River Parkway. It was dark and raining like hell, just pissing, and every car sent up a high spray as it raced by. Mum got more and more agitated as she strained on tiptoe to find a cab. Then a car turned out of the zoo on mum's blind side, whirled through a puddle and drenched her. At that moment my mother let rip a day's worth of frustration and anxiety, expressed in a single glorious outburst.

"FUCKING . . . SHIT!"

I cowered.

Geoff looked incredulous.

Soaked, angry, panicky, my mother corralled my cousin and me in dual headlocks and walked us more or less out into the middle of the road. She stood in front of an oncoming bus with her beloved son and nephew clutched to her side and she waited patiently for the driver to stop and open the door.

He did.

"Lady, whatayoudoin?"

"I'd like to get back downtown," she replied in a slightly strangled though still dignified Lower Canadian contralto, "and I'd like you to get us there . . . now."

Clutched in a side headlock that might have stymied Gene Kiniski, I clambered onto the bus and sat with my head jammed under mother's armpit. The bus drove us to a subway station. I seem to remember my mother asking a series of anxious questions, to which the driver answered repeatedly and good-naturedly, "Don't you worry, ma'am, we'll get youze dere. Don't you worry, we'll get youze where ya going."

We got on the subway and made our way down from the two hundreds towards midtown Manhattan. Across from us sat a man wearing a wide-brimmed powder blue fedora, working a toothpick back and forth in his mouth. I seem to remember that one of his two front teeth looked to be made of gold.

We had to change trains, and mum insisted that we form a human chain so as to fight our way through the crowds. Your average New York subway commuter, staggering through Penn Station on a late afternoon in mid-June 1972, was graced by the sight of my mother, jaw set, eyes narrow, bulling through the traffic like a charging offensive tackle, dragging two midgets behind her. She spoke hardly a word, and for all our protests she stared intently ahead of her, looking to keep us from being crushed by the surging crowds.

THE ACCIDENT

In matters touching on death, the clinical and the moral are never so far apart that we can look at one without seeing the other.

—SHERWIN B. NULAND, *How We Die*

All your life you think you have to hold back your craziness, but when you're sick you can let it out in all its garish colours.

—ANATOLE BROYARD, *Intoxicated by My Illness*

FOR ME, MEMORIES OF JUNE 10, 1974, start with breakfast. Later, when I threw it up in the emergency room, a nurse who was cutting my clothes away remarked how lucky I was to get scrambled eggs. "Those must have been delicious," she said cheerily.

It wasn't luck. It was habit. My dad, being a creature of military routine, served up the same breakfast every morning: eggs, half a grapefruit, two rashers of bacon, toast (no crust), juice and milk. The blue and white plate always sat on top of a solid placemat depicting an Audubon nature scene. The twelve- to fifteen-minute run of the meal was measured out by the sections of *The Globe and Mail*, each delivered to me as my dad finished them: front section (IN THE MIDST OF WATERGATE PRESIDENT NIXON PLANS TRIP TO MIDDLE EAST. 1400 GUESTS AT WHITE HOUSE RECEPTION CHANT "GOD BLESS NIXON!"), sports (a more or less straight report of the previous evening's wrestling card at Maple Leaf Gardens: SHEIK IS CARRIED OUT BUT STAYS UNDEFEATED), comics (*Blondie*, *Rex Morgan*, *Pogo*). Then he'd fold up the business section and march down the hall to the john for his "morning's morning." I'd saunter along behind, past the closing washroom door, a right turn into my room, loiter over something or other (*Sports Illustrated*, CFL player cards, Helmut Newton's latest shots in *Photo* magazine), pick up my knapsack and drop the rest of the paper off to my night-owl mother, still lolling in bed. Kiss goodbye, back past the john.

"See ya, dad."

"See ya, Sunny Jim."

On this day it was the same except that I left the house with only my history text attached to the back of my Raleigh ten-speed. I had an exam—Mr. Kidell's Grade 9 British history class. Two hours. I wasn't exactly full of confidence. I unlocked my bike, pulled my chain-side grey sock up over my grey flannel trouser leg, rolled the bike around to the front of our house and took off along Lonsdale Road towards Russell Hill. From there it was south past St. Clair Avenue, sailing all the way down the long hill that was the old Lake Iroquois shoreline, under the railway bridge to the corner of Dupont and Davenport. Then a right turn past Tony Sisca's Esso station, where my dad got his car gassed up (and where, as a result, I was able to gather extra Esso NHL power players), west along Dupont past Loblaws, past Spadina, negotiate the wiggle in that otherwise straight-arrow street, and left down Howland Avenue two long blocks to the Anglican boys' choir school, St. George's College, which I had attended for five years. Twenty more minutes to bone up, then bring on those Anglos and those Saxons. That was the plan.

I passed Loblaws in the warm morning light and approached the intersection of Spadina and Dupont. I was aware of a truck to my left, felt its steamy presence. I went past the passenger-side door, high over my left shoulder. The light was red, then it was green. Without a backward glance I started to walk the bike between my legs across the intersection. At the same moment, the truck started to turn right up Spadina. As it moved into me, I started to hop-waddle-walk, trying to turn with it, but now the bulk of the truck began exerting a gravitational force, drawing me and the bike inexorably under the rear wheel. I felt a steadily increasing pressure, and I remember a clear thought as the truck turned around me, my body falling gradually between the right rear tire, the curb and a lamp-post: "I'm in trouble." Then an odd thought: "This is what it would be like if I were mashed by the big freezer in our basement." There was a final crushing sensation and then the pavement, stretching away south down Spadina Avenue to the horizon, rose up and pounded me. I didn't fall to meet it, it rose to meet me, and it loomed there far and wide and black . . . blacker . . . blackest.

Then it was like waking up in the morning, a momentary sense that what had just happened might not really have happened. Next, someone—a policeman, as it turned out—was asking me questions. My eyes opened onto a huge du Maurier cigarette sign looming over me, and I responded in peppy rapid fire as much to reassure myself that everything was going to be fine as to satisfy the cop. I rattled off my name, address, phone number ("foureightsix-eighteenthirty") and parents' names ("Cicely'n'Norman"). I mentioned that I was going to be late for my history exam. Not that I thought this a negative thing—far from it. More time to study. I knew I was woefully ill prepared.

The cop laughed and said I wouldn't be writing anything any time soon.

"But I'm going to be okay, right?"

"Sure, probably a couple of broken ribs."

I don't remember any acute sensation of pain at that stage. As a precaution, I was lifted on a hard stretcher into an ambulance. I remember thinking that my back wasn't the problem. Shortly after the ambulance started to move the pain opened up like a blossom and I asked the attendant for something to kill it. No, he said, if we give you something, the doctors will have a more difficult time figuring out what's the matter.

By now the pain was like a pulsating sensation of white, everywhere inside me and all around me. It wasn't something that was happening to me. It *was* me. I kept asking where we were, as if my knowing would relieve the relentlessness of it all.

Then we were there—the Hospital for Sick Children. As I was wheeled into Emergency, I found myself cursing the truck driver, swearing a blue streak. "Fucking bastard, if I ever get my hands on that cocksucker . . ." I thought maybe I should be angry—after all, it was his fault, he had a truck, I had a bike, hardly a fair fight—so I was. A resident on the medical staff would later meet my mother in the waiting room and tell her, "Nice kid, but he's got a mouth on him like a stevedore." Meantime, the pain had subsided and I began to feel not better so much as not much at all. This, I'd later discover, is a clear indication of shock, the body's way of turning the pain volume down (and, unhappily, often a way station to the hereafter).

At this point, the unreliability of memory being what it is, my effort to recount the history of my trauma takes on a slightly more respectable cast. My medical records come into play, and the history of my accident and subsequent illness gets tied in with the efforts of those who succeeded in saving me.

On a clear spring day in 1996, my mother called me around to my parents' house on a leafy cul-de-sac in southeast Rosedale. Dad met me at the door, then disappeared. Mum was waiting in the living room, surrounded by shelf after shelf of eighteenth-century porcelain sauceboats. Her face is my face—a prominent jaw takes it past beautiful and nearer to handsome—a straight Roman nose, wide-apart and deep-set eyes. It's a mobile face, a face built for mimicry and mocking. She sat me down and told me—and these are her words—that she had "a spot of terminal cancer."

If my mother were to describe a mother and son exactly like us but not us, she'd point out that "they get along after a fashion"; in other words, war carried on by other means. Of course that's now, that's who we've become. When I was a little boy, my mother would read me C. S. Lewis's *The Lion, the Witch and the Wardrobe*, and by a flick of the eyebrow or a turn of the lip she could make me laugh or cry, sometimes on the same page, and for that I loved her unabashedly.

So when she said she was dying, I felt the craziest curry of thought and emotion. I wept, which is rare, and my mother said she didn't want me to feel badly. Then she told me she had recently tried to commit suicide. The way she described it, she walked out to the garage in her nightie and slippers with some duvets, pillows and a book of Cecil Beaton's photographs, shut the garage door, turned on the engine of dad's car, then curled up on the concrete floor in her duvets, with her Beaton, and fell asleep. "The only problem," she said, "was that your father's car ran out of gas."

We both laughed—first, because the situation was funny on its face and second, because dad's so scrupulous he never lets the car get below half a tank. Mum even added what I'm sure was an apocryphal grace note to her story, a confrontation with dad the next morning, a how-could-you-do-this-to-me? scene.

At that moment I thought I'd better tell my mother *how* I loved her. Just saying that I loved her wouldn't do; it would be exactly the sort of sentimental imprecision she and I mocked in others. I found myself thanking her for the way she had cared for me after the accident. And to the extent I could dole out the unconditional love so admired by therapists and preachers, that was it.

Later, walking home in the clear air, I noticed every blossom on every bush and tree, and I thought I better get on with writing an account of that accident or my mother would die and with her would go her crucial contribution to this story. I'd miss yet another opportunity to square myself with myself. I needed to understand and, by doing so, excise the accident and its aftermath. I needed a new way of thinking, one that didn't assume that the course of my illness was, and would always be, the course of my life.

The first step was to go over to Sick Kids and apply for the record of my hospitalization. Two weeks and seventy-five bucks later, I was sitting on a bench just outside the hospital's old front entrance on University Avenue, hungrily leafing through a five-inch stack of photocopies. I was surprised to find at the top a record of my tonsillectomy (November 25, 1963). It indicated that I weighed 39 1/4 pounds and had ginger ale shortly after the operation. I remember the strange sensation of waking up in the evening light, the feel of vanilla ice cream running down my throat. I looked for that on the chart. Not there.

And then I saw it: my admission record for June 10, 1974. "Multiple trauma," it read. From there it was a litany of medical terminology chronicling my ups and downs (the progress report), a record of every order given by the doctors charged with my care, and technical reports indicating the results of a variety of blood tests. As I read, I became increasingly discouraged by the distance between what I'd felt and what they had written. For instance, one passage referred to draining 5.7 litres of fluid from my abdomen. That's it—one declarative sentence. Having 5.7 litres of fluid drained from your abdomen, I thought, deserves more telling than that.

In fact, in pursuing the story of my illness, I sensed that all these events deserved more telling. It's certainly how I felt at the time. I wanted to tell people what was happening to me, but doctors and nurses and friends and relations and parents weren't all that interested in letting me talk (or at least in listening to me), because I was sick unto death and the big thing was to make me better. I remember as I left the emergency room on my way to the intensive care unit, my dad, six foot two in a crisply pressed grey-checked suit, a pansy affixed to his lapel as always, suddenly appearing beside my gurney as it rolled towards the elevator. Like most teenagers who've screwed up, I needed to explain myself. So, as was—and is—my wont, I babbled nervously about who knows what. Dad looked down and pleaded with me to keep quiet and save my energy. And I actually remember being pissed off. *He never lets me talk.*

I suppose, in some still-adolescent fashion, I want to talk now just as I did then. To speak my mind about my illness and my mother's cancer. What that might amount to, I don't know. My mind has been resistant to pattern and sense as long as I can remember. I'm all for stumbling blind down the alley.

As a practical matter, the accident stayed with me by way of a series of acute pancreatic illnesses in 1977, 1987 and 1990, each resulting in extended stays in the hospital. In a more abstract sense, the guy I wake up to be every day is, for better or worse, the guy who got run over by a truck; the scars deeply embedded in my midsection always remind me. Nervous dad, nervous writer, nervous guy. Me. Every so often I meet someone from the small circle of old-money WASP Toronto in which I was raised, and we'll do the "oh-do-you-know-so-and-so?" waltz. Inevitably it will be interrupted by "Oh, you're the guy that got run over by the truck." Blood, bile, pus, puke, scars, stitches, Demerol, IV needles, sodium pentothal, catheters, nasogastric tubes, laparotomy and jejunostomy, and every other goddamn thing that happened to me that summer and subsequently—more than anything else, I am that guy.

At any rate, before I could hope to address these matters, I had to go back and reconstruct things. Apart from my medical records, I figured the best place to begin would be with my parents and the doctors who treated me. With one major exception, the main players were still around. Dr. Sigmund Ein, who'd been responsible for my case while the surgeon in charge was on vacation, still practised general surgery at Sick Kids. Dr. Mark Greenberg, a medical resident at the time, was now head of pediatric oncology. I remembered him as a decent fellow, often willing to talk *to* me as opposed to talking *about* me. Dr. Adelaide Fleming, my pediatrician at the time, was also still practising. All agreed to see me.

The exception was Dr. Clinton Stephens, the senior surgeon in charge of my case, who had died of cancer in April 1990. My mum and I had gone to a memorial service at Timothy Eaton church. As we left, she turned to me and said, "Well, that was a good deed in a dirty world." I had the vague feeling that I'd missed something by not keeping in touch with Dr. Stephens through the years. In a tribute published in the *Journal of Pediatric Surgery*, Dr. Ein and two others in the department of general surgery wrote: "He was a precise, gentle, definitive technical surgeon, and always taught conservative surgery. His patient care was simple, easy, and impeccable. His knowledge of pediatric surgery was encyclopedic; his recall for patients and their problems was both accurate and uncanny."

In short, he was pretty much as heroic as I remembered him. Speaking laconically if at all, Dr. Stephens radiated a kind of charismatic calm. He would always ask how I was doing and I was always ready with a report that would daunt a royal commission. As I spoke, he would palpate my belly with his large callused hands in a manner that I found immensely reassuring. I would prattle on and he would respond, "Uh hhuuuh, hmmmhh, uh huh." Then he would check my chest with his always chilly stethoscope, look down with amused blue eyes set wide beneath a high patrician forehead, and say, "We'll come by again a little later." And off he would go, a gaggle of sober residents and interns trailing behind his slow certain gait.

The record of my first day in the hospital indicates that, as a general observation, my condition was "pale, clammy, apprehensive, conversant, cooperative, intelligent," which from the sounds of it is me most days. (If only that last observation meant something more than its clinical definition, "having or showing understanding.") The more specific notations were really quite encouraging. Despite abrasions on my right face and right orbit, there was no "boney [sic] tenderness." Despite "rapid respiration" and "a slight paradoxical movement of the left sternum" (indicative, I discovered later, of a punctured lung) there was no "lateral chest tenderness." And, wonder of wonders, under the heading "Genit" were the words every fourteen-year-old boy, whether he knows it or not, longs to see: "normal male."

Reading my charts for June 10, 1974, it looked to me as if I was a slightly overwrought kid aiming to please. Of course, it was all much worse than that. My blood pressure when I entered the emergency room was 80/0, my pulse was 140, my respiration 60 and shallow. Together, these three readings represented a physical catastrophe in the making. My heart whacking away at over twice its normal rate was compensating for severe internal bleeding. Losing the blood was starving the brain of oxygen, so the brain responded by trying to up the intake. But the punctured lung restricted the power of my bellows. Hence my breaths were as shallow as the shoreline. As for my blood pressure, well, any time a zero shows up in the reading it's cause for concern. I was a mess. Just how much of a mess was made clear to me in two sobering exchanges, with Doctors Ein and Fleming.

I caught up with Dr. Ein, who bears a striking resemblance to the U.S. federal reserve chairman, Alan Greenspan, at Sick Kids.

His office is an event in itself. There are photographs everywhere, mostly of doctors standing around at medical gatherings. Balloons and streamers hang from the ceiling and litter the floor. Bumper stickers, diplomas and a Michael Jordan mask plaster the walls. Draped across the back of his chair is Hulk Hogan's torn tank top, signed.

During my stay at the hospital I found out that he and his wife, an ICU nurse at the hospital, had adopted six kids, all of whom Dr. Ein had operated on. I remembered two things about his manner: first, while moving around my bed during an examination, his head swivelled like that of an agitated turtle; and second, he brushed off my questions in a manner meant to discourage any further queries. At one point, during the month he was charged with my care, he actually restricted me to two questions per visit. "Make 'em count," he said. I asked him which was his favourite baseball team. "Cincinnati Reds," he said without missing a beat. "That's one."

In my interview with Dr. Ein, I tried to get a sense of exactly what had happened to me that morning twenty-four years earlier. I remembered the term *hematoma* being bandied about.

"A hematoma's a big bruise," Ein said. "It's like if I give you a big smash in the arm. I'll burst the blood vessels, and bust the muscle, and you bleed into it and you get a hematoma. The liver's got a very fragile capsule that, if you give a good shock to it, it'll break." Dr. Ein's eyes grew wide as his explanation gathered momentum. "Have you ever seen raw liver? Take your fist, next time you see it, before your mom cooks it, and pound it like this"—he smashed his fist on his desktop, BANG—"and it'll tear apart. And that's exactly what your liver looked like." It occurred to me that the chances of my mother cooking liver for me were... remote. I managed, however, to keep this thought to myself.

Later that week I went to speak with Dr. Fleming at her home office on Dunvegan Avenue in Forest Hill, just around the corner from where I'd grown up. Once inside the door I was hit by a smell I remembered exactly, a powerful combination of disinfectant and eucalyptus. Dr. Adelaide Fleming shared the same comfortable, WASPy background as my mother. She was puzzled as to what exactly I was up to. "Why do you want to explore this in such detail?" she asked. "I mean, the detail of the operations and your course in the hospital. I could see how you could write, say, about the powerful influence this had on you psychologically, but I'm surprised you want to relive the agony."

I ventured something about resembling a litigant who wants to inform himself of all the details so he can make a persuasive argument, but I'm not even sure I bought that myself. Then we got down to it.

"I remember that those first few days were very intense. Stephens wasn't very happy with the situation."

"When you say he wasn't very happy," I asked, suddenly wishing I was very far away, "what do you mean?"

Her face became calm, matter-of-fact. "Well, he thought you were going to die; that's what he kept telling me. I was more optimistic. I felt that if we could just keep you supported you'd be all right."

Right then I had a clear recollection of asking my mother whether I was going to die. She was sitting bedside on one of those first few days. She turned her profile to me and said, "No, you're going to get better. You're very, very ill, but you're going to get better." (Unbeknownst to me, my mother had by this time already written my obituary for inclusion in *The Globe and Mail* should the need arise.) As she spoke, she looked out the window, up and away across University Avenue, maybe catching a corner of the newly minted Mount Sinai Hospital across the street.

I'd always known that I had been very sick. I probably even knew that I'd almost died. But hearing that Dr. Stephens believed I *would* die . . .

Dr. Fleming continued to speak, but it was as though she were moving away from me down a long tunnel. I could see that she was talking, but her words weren't reaching me.

Because of the "extensive disruption of the right lobe of the liver," blood, bile, tissue fluid and intravenous fluid poured out of my liver into my abdominal cavity. As a result my abdomen increased several waist sizes, to 86 centimetres in girth from the regular 62. I remember the nurses coming in every hour or so and measuring. I couldn't even lift my rump to let them pass the tape measure under my back. I learned just what the word "distended" means. The sensation is unpleasant in the extreme. Push out your abdomen as though you're trying to create the impression you have a bowling ball lodged in your gut. Push hard; strain until your belly starts to quiver. Now hold that position for seventy-two hours and you'll have some sense of how it felt.

I noticed on the charts that in these early days they were giving me doses of Valium, presumably to keep me in a relaxed state. Because of my immobility, nurses would come and beat gently on my chest to make me cough to keep fluid from gathering in my lungs. The record says that I developed pneumonia. Within two or three days I was severely jaundiced, my skin turning lime green as my liver failed to remove pollutants from the bloodstream. I remember the whites of my eyes turning the shade of egg yolk.

The ruptured liver, as it turned out, wasn't the problem. The fluid pouring out was. "Once you were stabilized and on intravenous, and the blood was starting to transfuse, the chances of you dying from that injury were pretty small," said Dr. Ein. "After that, however, bile and blood mixed together in the belly, and the risk of infection was significant—especially when this stuff stays in your belly. It stays in an area or pocket that's stagnant, just like water in a pool. There's no circulation, and it pollutes, and organisms grow very well in blood and bile. They're very nutritious."

In other words I was a prime candidate for septic shock, the leading cause of "late death" (death days or weeks following trauma) in ICU patients. Septic shock is a deadly chain reaction triggered by the infection to which Dr. Ein referred. One organ fails and the rest follow along, like so many horses pulling the hearse.

To remedy this situation Dr. Siran Bandy, a poker-faced East Indian, turned up at my bedside five days after the accident, inserted an angiocatheter no. 14 into my right side and proceeded to withdraw 5.7 litres of fluid from my abdomen. (There are, in fact, only around 5 litres of blood in a fourteen-year-old boy's entire body.) Down the length of my trunk I could see the maroon liquid running out of me the way water flows freely from an outdoor tap. Now and again Dr. Bandy mopped his brow. The stuff reeked. At that moment I began to feel myself changing from a guy who'd experienced something like a bad cut or abrasion to someone else. "Look at all that shit pouring out of me," I thought, and for whatever reason I found it funny. I tried to say something to Dr. Bandy about how weird it was to have a spigot punched in my side, draining all that crap from my body. His dark eyes stared back at me over his face mask. "I'll be finished soon," he said.

I like to think that in those moments I was taking the first baby steps towards developing what Anatole Broyard called a "style" for my sickness. "I think," Broyard wrote in *Intoxicated by My Illness*, a posthumously published chronicle of his mortal bout with prostate cancer, "that only by insisting on your style can you keep from falling out of love with yourself as the illness attempts to diminish or disfigure you. Sometimes your vanity is the only thing that keeps you alive, and your style is the instrument of your vanity. It may not be dying we fear so much, but the diminished self."

The degree of my diminishment was very much on my medical team's mind in those first few days. There was, in fact, a delicate minuet being danced by the doctors. Dr. Ein remembered there being "a lot of pressure that you should be operated on right away." Dr. Stephens, however, disagreed and solicited a consultation from a senior surgeon at the Toronto General to support him in what Dr. Ein described as his "conservative approach."

Other surgeons would have acted much more quickly to remove the damaged part of the liver. But in my case the damage was so extensive—"such a big mushy thing," as

Dr. Ein put it—that Dr. Stephens decided to proceed "non-operatively," at least for the first couple of weeks. (This course of action has since become much more the rule in treating massive liver damage.) If he expected me to die anyway, I'd like to think that in pursuing this course Dr. Stephens was executing a bold two-part plan. First, he was doing no harm, which, as my later experience with medical care would demonstrate, is the true genius of medical practice. Second, he was leaving room for a miracle.

A week after the maple-tree tap job, with a further 2.6 litres of fluid having been drained from my abdomen, I was taken into surgery, where I had drainage tubes inserted above and below the damaged portion of the liver. I read in the surgical notes that I was returned to the ICU after the operation on June 22 in "fairly good shape." I remember waking up and having no idea whether it was day or night and wishing that this would all be over.

As the days went by, my chances got steadily better. The leakage from the liver diminished and the cocktails of antibiotics and nutritional supplements began to take hold. The arrows scattered throughout my progress notes started turning in the right direction. Hemoglobin, blood pressure, respiration, pulse, all to the good.

There's a photograph of me taken during this period. A nasogastric tube is attached to my face by two pieces of white tape that cross my upper lip and forehead. An oxygen mask, removed for the photograph, sits on top of my head. My right arm is taped up like a ball player's from elbow to wrist and thrown rakishly over my head, which if I remember correctly was the only comfortable way of holding it. My left arm rests by my side, similarly taped, with a blood pressure cuff affixed above the elbow. What

I'd forgotten was that in addition to the IVs in my arm I had an IV that ran directly into my jugular vein. The sheet is pulled up over my stomach. I'm smiling. On the whole I look like an actor playing a sick teen in a medical drama.

It is at this point that Dr. Mark Greenberg's remarks start showing up in my records. He was the only doctor who made reference to me by name. His first entry is dated June 26, 1974. In his careful script, on a single line at the top of a page, he wrote, "Douglas looks better today." For whatever reason I felt enlivened whenever he came around.

I managed to elicit a one-hour interview with Dr. Greenberg in his office at Sick Kids. Given that his secretary has him scheduled at fifteen-minute intervals, that was a coup. He's among the most sought-after cancer consultants in the world, and his time is, in a very real sense, precious. He was just as I remembered him, a tall, toothy, gangly South African. His face broke into a huge grin when he saw me.

"I never expected one of my former patients to come see me at age forty-one," he said.

I couldn't help myself. "I'm actually thirty-eight."

The smile faded slightly. Did he remember meeting and talking with me? "My sense was, by the time I came in contact with you, you had progressed to the point where you had a severe but not life-threatening illness. You had gone from an acute to a long-term chronic problem." How did he know it was potentially a long-term problem? "Because the location of the injury was around the pancreatic duct and the pancreatic head. I understand you have a history of obstruction around that area. You were a candidate for that condition. That was one of my concerns in treating you."

Really? Then why the hell didn't anybody mention that to me at the time? And why was it that each time I had a pancreatic attack—four over the next sixteen years—nobody ever linked the pancreatitis to my accident, even though one of those attacks came as close to killing me as the truck did? No, they all opted for medicine's favourite free pass, referring to my attacks as "idiopathic," meaning "arising spontaneously or from an unknown cause."

I managed to hold my anger in check and asked Dr. Greenberg what he recalled about perking me up. "I remember talking to you when you took a nosedive—emotionally frustrated and depressed—sitting and chatting to you."

I suddenly recalled something about his having had an accident as a kid. I asked him about it. "I had an injury playing squash. We actually talked about it. I had a head injury and had to have a craniotomy. I was very sick after, so I had a perspective on what it was like to be sick. I have often talked about the term that applies to sick people—*invalid*—as deriving very concretely from the words that comprise it: *in valid.* Becoming dependent or being dependent is particularly hard for young males."

I asked if he remembered the course of my depression. "As I remember, you were very sick, though quite bouncy and cheery, and then became less sick and less bouncy. I kept coming to talk to you after I was no longer responsible for your medical care. Fourteen and dealing with an illness, that's difficult—too old for Mother Goose and too young for Kafka. Fourteen-year-olds are moving forward developmentally; they get sick, they regress, and you're left with this sort of boy-man. You were in a twilight zone. If you know you're never going to get better, you have to come to terms with a new reality. Your problem was the uncertainty. I don't know why it's so vivid in my memory of you that you were not self-correcting; you were confused. The hard part was that you weren't quite sure where the end would be. I think that's what you were thinking."

After that interview I was both heartened and put off—heartened because Dr. Greenberg had been the kind of doctor who treated *me* as opposed to my condition, and put off because I hadn't been quite the laugh-in-the-face-of-adversity mensch I'd always thought. Especially after I left the ICU for the first time on July 9, I saw myself cracking wise twenty-four hours a day. I remember watching the movie *M*A*S*H* and identifying with the characters played by Elliott Gould and Donald Sutherland. "I'm a pro from Dover too," I thought. I'd always seen the wise-cracking as countering my sense of physical diminution, which was pretty much ongoing. I also began to see how the course of my life had been dictated by the "boy-man" stepping out into the world for a moment, then back behind the folds of his mother's skirts (or the skirts of any woman that would have him), feeling safe or satisfied in neither place.

A couple of days after I saw Dr. Greenberg, I picked up some photo albums at my parents' house. I hadn't seen any pictures of myself from that period in a long time. There they were: shots from 1971 to 1974. Two from the fall of '74 were awful to contemplate. In one, my smile seems attached with staples and my eyes belong in formaldehyde. In the other, except for the acne, I look nine. As I studied them, I flashed back to a moment when I regarded myself in the mirror of my hospital room, shortly after the worst of the danger had passed but with a month or so still left in my incarceration. My ribs were sticking out of me like a med school skeleton. My neck looked like a flower stalk holding up a bowling ball. I turned away. I'm not sick, I'm ugly. There were gorgeous nurses everywhere, gorgeous, healthy, strong, vibrant women. I watched them, and though I knew they were caring for me, I feared that somewhere in the back of their mind they were thinking, "That poor, ugly, skinny bastard."

So I joked. I teased all the time—or at least all the time I wasn't *depressed*. I did imitations of Dr. Ein's turtle-headed manner, the residents, the priests and ministers who came around looking to save a lost soul. I made the nurses laugh. I owned them. I killed them. They're helpless when they're laughing. That was the style of my illness. I was fragile and ugly, but I was funny. And that, at least for a few seconds at a time, made me powerful.

My relationship with my parents was altogether different. With them it was a lot tougher to get any traction. I was their only son, my mother's only child. Mum, I remember, was a constant presence, first thing in the morning till late at night, looking out for me every way she knew how. Our relationship was complicated by my mother's desire to, well, mother me. All she saw was a very sick child who needed her constant attention. The jokes, the imitations, the barbs were lost on her. This was not because she didn't have a sense of humour; she could be hilarious. But her whole will, and it was considerable, was tuned to making me well, when in fact there wasn't much she could do about it. Still, she had to believe there was *something*.

She brought little pillows, big pillows, down-filled pillows and pillows for the small of my back. She bought special foods when I could eat, any books I wanted (the entire James

Bond series, which, in retrospect, must have nearly killed her). She organized my friends and relatives to come and see me. When I was too tired, she read to me: reams of get-well cards (not from my friends so much as her friends and friends of friends), *Sports Illustrated*, Bond, the comics from the British kids' magazine *Look and Learn*. She even read me the report of a football game as it appeared in the *Toronto Sun*, a newspaper I'm quite sure she had never opened before. When I was well enough, she would wheel me outside into a small courtyard behind the old nurses' residence, where we would tilt our exhausted faces towards the sun.

Mum worried about all the things she couldn't control. The doctor's mental health, for instance. Many years later Mum revealed to me that shortly before my accident the daughter of a great friend had conceived an illegitimate child with the son of one of my doctors. "Now all this burst on my unsuspecting brain in early July [three weeks after the accident]. It does affect one in a funny way. You find that someone with whom you thought you were going to have a totally impersonal relationship...you just aren't." Whether any of this is true, and whether it coloured his thinking, is beside the point. My mother had been stepmother to a daughter who'd given birth to a child under complicated circumstances. At the time she had felt the stinging, unspoken disapprobation of her social peers, and she assumed that the doctor must feel something similar. The thought that shook her to her soul was that he would sense that she knew all this and that, somehow, this would affect his treatment of me. All of this remained unspoken, though it was plain across twenty-five years that the thought of some begrudging on the doctor's part that affected his treatment of her child still terrified my mother. As a result of all this, I suspect, mum was capable of almost superhuman identification with, and protection of, children in distress.

One time she was in the hospital lounge smoking a cigarette to keep herself sane. A woman and her young son were also there presumably to visit a sick relative. Mum hadn't noticed them at first, as she sucked the smoke gratefully down to the farthest reaches of her lungs, holding it there for a second before releasing it through her nose and then her mouth in a prolonged sigh. Just then the woman slapped the child. "You shuddup. You siddown." Mum was up in a split second, towering over the woman, her features puffed with a gargantuan rage. "Don't you touch one hair on that child's head. I won't allow it." The woman shot something back. The boy looked confused. Mother remonstrated loudly enough to bring in a passing nurse to investigate. The woman and the child scurried out, leaving my quivering mother alone in the room.

As for my dad, it's a much shorter story. He came every day at noon on the dot for half an hour, walking up from his office at King and Bay, a yard to the stride, fifteen minutes to the mile, as certain as sunlight. In the evening he would return to collect mum and stay another half-hour. His job was clear. Like the composed officer under fire at Ortona, he deployed his emotional resources to ensure a successful campaign. He rarely referred to my illness directly, preferring to ask, "How are things?" I would always reply, "Better." He seemed full of confidence and power. At the time, he was chairman of Sunnybrook Hospital, which he had helped transform from a veterans' care hospital into an acute care hospital. Tall, cool and commanding, he scared the nurses, and I got treated with a good deal more deference whenever he was around.

At one point he told me that he had gone through his war and now I was going through mine. This is truer than I knew at the time, for he had been wounded at Ortona, losing some of his left arm and chest. He was hopitalized on Malta for four months, waiting for skin grafts to take hold—they didn't—then got malaria followed by more skin grafts, and on and on. I once asked what he remembered of the experience. "There was an Irish nurse who brought me a bottle of Carling Black Label beer, which was actually vermouth. Beyond that . . . it was just dull."

Knowledge of my father's history made me believe in him in a way that his aloof stoicism never did. In the summer of 1995, on the anniversary of VE day, I did a radio commentary for the CBC in which I talked about how my dad had never let me down that summer, "not even once." What I didn't mention was that I let him down *more* than once, mostly by bitching at mum for embarrassing me in front of the nurses. Dad would scold me right on the spot—a cold look, a curt "Pipe down," followed by something about "having to help mum get through all this." Dad viewed illness with a cold realist's eye. It's an interregnum: get over it and move on.

There's a photograph of me and my cousin Geoff Scott taken at the cottage the summer after my accident. I look healthier but still painfully thin. I seem to remember that I had my shirt off just before the picture was taken and that dad insisted I keep it off for the photo. I remember angry tears springing from my eyes as I refused his badgering requests. But I knew he meant well, so, as best I could, I swallowed the humiliation I felt, lump after lump, down my gullet to a place where rage sits for a lifetime.

On July 30, having recently suffered a severe fever and considerable weight loss, I was operated on by Dr. Stephens and a team of six assistants. In a six-hour procedure, they rewired my entire digestive system, hooking my stomach directly to my bowel to bypass the damaged duodenum, drained several abscesses, and inserted a feeding tube directly into my belly. I was readmitted to the ICU in a segregated area designed to prevent post-operative infection. The room was glassed in. I had no contact with the other patients but could see and hear them through the glass walls. At night the place was full of electronic bleeps and blips emanating from various monitors tracking heart and respiration rates and regulating the flow of intravenous fluids. Every so often the darkness was pierced by the harrowing sound of a child in deep distress. Every so often, it was me.

In the room next to mine was a young girl, eight, maybe nine years old. She was dying. On several occasions alarms rang in her room and a team of doctors and nurses would rush to revive her. Each time I looked over at her, she was either unconscious or gasping for air. When her parents visited, they brought balloons and other little knickknacks. Then they would sit by the bed and hold on to each other. The mother often reached out to stroke her daughter's dark brown hair or caress her cheek.

One day the catheter in my penis started to bother me, so I asked the nurse if she could either remove it or in some other way make me comfortable. She replied that it would take at least two nurses to deal with my problem and that everybody else was tied up next door. "Why do you bother?" I heard myself asking. "She's going to die anyway." The nurse, her back to me, shuddered and spun round. "How can you say that?" she asked with genuine disgust. The enormity of my selfishness struck me, and after a couple of feeble apologies I shut up.

However tempted I might be to moralize retrospectively on this incident, the brute fact remains that the will to live trumps whatever feeble efforts I might make to either justify or condemn my own behaviour. The little girl died and I lived. It's as simple as that. Or maybe it's not as simple as that. Some part of me longs to believe I deserved to live precisely because another part of me suspects I deserved to die.

Ten days after the operation I suffered what amounted to a heart attack. I had managed to get out of bed for one of the first times since the surgery. It had taken two nurses to move me three feet from the bed to the chair. I had just settled in and was working a Laura Secord sucker (green, I think) when my heart suddenly began to gallop. "Oh shit," I said, "oh fuck, my heart's going too fast."

In a moment my mother was right in front me. "Douglas, what's wrong? Are you choking on that sucker?" What she really intended was more of a command: "Stop choking on that sucker." Whenever my mother panicked, she was always hit by a mix of rage and fear. Her expression changed in the same way: she drew her cheeks in and bit down hard on the flesh on the inside of her mouth. It never failed to provoke me into a similar rage. She was looking at me that way now, as I struggled to get air into my lungs.

"Are you choking on the sucker?"

"No," I said, my voice rising, "I'm not choking on the fucking sucker." As my heart raced to nowhere, I winged that lollipop with everything I had. It shattered on the porcelain sink over on the other side of the room. Suddenly, nurses and doctors were all around me, placing an oxygen mask over my mouth and nose, taking an electrocardiogram. I kept asking if I was having a heart attack. One of the residents, Dr. David Hitch, a drawling, po-faced Carolinian, answered, "Yeaaassss, it's possible." Dr. Mark Bleisher, his fellow resident, asked him in a stern voice to step outside, where I've always hoped he pounded Hitch's brains out through his ears. I felt my eyes roll back in fear and panic, and just at that moment I caught my mother's eye. "You see," I thought, "you can't *wish* this shit away, can you?"

My "progress" report for that day noted that I was readmitted to the ICU and that I'd had a pulmonary embolism (a blockage in the artery), "although there was definitely a component of anxiety state in the patient's response." In subsequent years this anxiety state played out again and again like a leitmotif. One time, when I thought I was having a heart attack, I staggered out into traffic in front of several thousand dog racing fans, my pants falling around my knees, along the main highway between Palm Beach and Fort Lauderdale.

Even so, and knowing all my subsequent history, I was still put off as I read the doctor's description of my "anxious" behaviour of August 1974. "Fuck off," I thought. "You try having a pulmonary embolism in front of your mother."

One evening following my heart troubles I was wheeled down to the X-ray department. It was a recurring feature of my recovery: a series of X-rays to track the improving condition of my innards. On this occasion the late summer sun was dropping beneath the horizon and the building was suffused in a fading pink light. I was greeted by an expressionless technician who in the usual manner moved me against one wall to position me. He placed his hands on my shoulders to square me up. I felt his hands against my bones. His thumbs pressed against my clavical. For a second it hurt. As he held me there, he said, "You're too skinny." The charts indicate that I weighed somewhere between 80 and 100 pounds.

It's hard to imagine this remark was meant to be wounding. It was an observation probably meant in a sort of cajoling, lighthearted fashion, though for the life of me I can't remember anything in his tone to indicate this. In any event, I was mortified. I was on the edge of puberty and in one fell swoop I'd lost any confidence whatsoever in my body. And though it sounds melodramatic, in some ways I would never get it back.

Shortly before I started writing this book, I went to see mum to collect her memories of my illness. She was bedridden, her left arm a big bag of cancer wrapped in dressings and bandages changed twice a day by a Victorian Order nurse. She was tired and her eyes drooped under the influence of painkillers. But twenty-four years after that miserable summer, her clawing, snapping, snarling will was still on display.

We started out discussing chronology.

"On July the ninth, I was let out back up to—"

"The survival unit."

"No, no, I went onto a ward."

"That's what I call a survival unit."

"Why?"

"Because, as far as I was concerned, that's what it was. There was no care, no attention, no nothin'. You were lucky you survived."

"Right, well, there were some good nurses and there were some bad nurses."

"There were some really bad nurses, really bad. I mean, they had no training. They knew nothing from nothing. Ignorant peasants is what they were."

I tried to get her off this, but she wouldn't quit.

"Did they hate me, boy oh boy, oh boy, did they hate me, and I hated them. You know what they used to say to you? The darling things, they would go and see you in the morning before you got out of bed, before you woke up, and say, 'You'll never be part of this floor because she's so neurotic.'"

Christ, I thought, she's right. They did say that stuff.

"I mean, such bitches, such bitches I could not believe. I did it their way or I didn't do it at all. And they did it wrong quite a lot of the time. I'm not making that up."

"What sort of things?"

"They wouldn't turn up on time, turn up with your medicines on time. They were careless and stupid and overbearing."

"Mother—"

"Those women were beyond description."

"Yeah, well—"

"Cruel, wicked, evil, vile, filthy creatures."

I asked mum if she was sure those were the words she wanted on the permanent record.

"I can use some more if you like."

"No," I said, laughing, "I think that will do nicely, thank you."

Mum's vitriol belied a complex and subtle attitude towards those who cared for me. Every year since the accident she'd taken an enormous fancy-food basket and left it for the ICU staff working through the night on Christmas Eve. Some of the nurses on that shift were infants at the time of my accident. Like much that powered my mother's life, it was an act born of both gratitude and obligation. Irrespective of the bile she'd just let loose, the simple fact remains—I was saved—and, duty bound, my mum went every Christmas Eve to thank those responsible.

Mum flagged, her eyes dropping shut. I touched her good hand and wandered out of the bedroom thinking that, whatever I might write about my experiences and my mother's role in them—good, bad or indifferent—no matter how embarrassed she made me, her fearsome, angry, ineffable love is like gravity. So long as I'm walking around, my steps rise and fall with hers.

Lately, my mum's been getting worse. I go to see her at my parents' new apartment overlooking Allan Gardens and the church steeples on Jarvis Street. There's an absorbent pad resting beneath her bottom. A walker sits beside the bed. I find it hard to visit her. We talk on the phone all the time, but going to see her is another matter. I'm often impatient, picking up copies of *The Spectator* that are strewn around her bed, wandering about, looking at her books, picking up the *petits objets* my mother has collected over her lifetime: fancy perfume bottles, silver snuff boxes, porcelain Limoges boxes where she keeps her stamps, a small stone box with an inlaid mother-of-pearl flower pattern on the lid.

She's wasting away to nothing and there's nothing I can do about it. When I get back home, I'm often irritable. I snap at my wife and ignore the kids. I steal away upstairs to watch television because, as an occasional television critic, "that's my job."

But I'm going to do better. I've promised my wife I'll stop yelling in front of the children, and I've promised myself that, no matter the circumstances, I'm going to go see mum at least three times a week till the end. And I'm going to sit and listen and try to be entertaining and engaging in a way she would appreciate. She has it coming.

As my mother lay dying, I still wondered: am I really, at the core, the guy who got run over by that truck or am I finally past that? This question had never occurred to me before.

When our kids bellyache about what they're eating for breakfast, lunch or dinner, my juridical wife whips out a terrific admonition that clams them up every time: "You get what you get." What I like about this bit of home wisdom is that it in no way vitiates free will or any of the other helpful illusions that get us up in the morning. It simply suggests that once the cards are dealt, you might as well get on with the game. And though I've promised myself to do a better job of living up to that sentiment, I also know even that's not enough. I need a way forward.

Later, I thought about that basket my mother took to the ICU every year at Christmas. Pretty soon someone else will have to take it. It might as well be me.

TEENAGER

After a day or two my funk blew away, leaving me clear and ready again for anything. I was an idiot, but I had reserves of courage and optimism that amaze me now.

—RICHARD RAYNER, *The Blue Suit*

AFTER LEAVING THE HOSPITAL on September 10, 1974, I spent four months at home and the rest of that school year attending half-days. Early on I remember feeling weak and helpless. A month or so after my release I went across the street to watch my would-a-, could-a-, should-a-been teammates play Upper Canada College. Someone passed a soccer ball towards me. It felt more like a medicine ball as it landed against my foot, and I could barely kick it back. I remember late fall afternoons eating lunch while watching Ginger Rogers and Fred Astaire swirl about the television in movies like *Flying Down to Rio*, *Top Hat*, *Shall We Dance* and *Swing Time*. I absolutely adored these movies. Astaire's easy athleticism spoke of a man utterly at home in his own skin.

My mother hired an English nanny to help out with my care. I was still very weak, and mum didn't like me walking the streets alone, ever. The nanny was pockmarked and haggish, with a literal mind and no discernible sense of humour. Dad and I immediately began plotting to get rid of her. This was mostly unspoken. Dad arranged his life so that anything the nanny was supposed to do, he would do first ("Oh, that's all right, we've already had breakfast, taken out the garbage, cleaned the silver and gutted the fish. Thank you!"). Or else he actively dissuaded her from doing something my mother had left strict instructions for her to do. ("There's no need to take the dog to the vet for his operation. No reason we can't do it right here.")

I added my own exquisite tortures. On my sojourns I forced the nanny to walk several paces behind me. If I happened to run into anyone I knew, there would be a horribly awkward scene. At a minimum, good form forced me to introduce her, leaving open the question of why she was following along behind me. In the event, I didn't even bother explaining that. Meanwhile the poor woman was forced to stand mute, her own repressed nanny ways holding her tongue in check.

Mum, of course, soon cottoned on to our wretched behaviour and would have none of it. "I cannot manage," she said, her voice full of exasperation and drama, "*this* household without extra help and besides, I am *utterly, utterly* exhausted."

I remember one time the nanny offered to make tea for my mother. "Yes, that would be lovely," mum replied, clearly enjoying the small luxury of this offer. "Dear," she said absently to me, tugging on her needlepoint, "could you ask the nanny for milk and sugar." I popped my head in the swinging kitchen door. "Milk and sugar if you don't mind." I came back to mum and a moment later the nanny appeared with the tea. On the tray were teacups and saucers and a glass of milk. The nanny withdrew and mother and I were left to look and wonder. It was what it appeared to be—a glass of milk with a heaping tablespoon of sugar thrown in. A perfectly literal execution of my request. Whether this was abject stupidity or a thumping repudiation of my bad behaviour remains an open question. Either way, the nanny was gone two weeks later.

At Eastertime in 1975 my mother organized a trip to Florida for me and my twin cousin, Geoff. We were to stay at La Coquille, a private club south of Palm Beach, with my mother and her parents, Douglas and Jesse Ambridge. My grandfather and namesake was a big bowl-backed fellow a shade over six feet tall and well over two hundred pounds. He was in his middle seventies by then and in a bad way thanks to lung cancer and alcoholism. He still had the air of menace about him that must have served him well as co-captain of the McGill university football team and later as an artillery gunner during the First World War. After that war he became a captain of industry who served during the next war as director of shipbuilding—one of C.D. Howe's dollar-a-year men—and went on from there to Abitibi-Price.

As seven-year-olds, Geoffrey and I had sat on his knees and had our picture taken at a family compound near St. Andrews. I remember early mornings marching out into the New Brunswick woods with my hand entombed in his. My memory of him belies his reputation (in *The Canadian Establishment*, Peter Newman referred to him as a "bombastic engineer"). He struck me as playful, even mischievous. He called us his little two-by-fours. There was something both powerful and exotic about him. Often he would break into Spanish (his first language) and laugh uproariously at the confused looks this brought to our faces. He'd been born and raised in Mexico City, the son of expatriate Canadians. His father, Charles, had made a killing in the mining business. (Family lore had it that my grandfather's brother, Teddy, had rebelled against his father's staunchly conservative ways and run off, only to be killed in some sort of mining explosion in Peru.)

As we drove to La Coquille from the Miami airport, my grandfather looked across the low Florida prospect and said, his voice as flat and grainy as sandpaper, "I hate this fucking place. Why are we here?" My mother and grandmother assumed expressions meant to indicate their displeasure, which might have registered with my grandpa except for one small impediment: he didn't give a damn.

During our stay I swam in a blue pool under the ever clear sky. I went to a driving range and swatted a bucket of balls. The golf clubs felt heavy and awkward, and my shots fluttered weakly, travelling only half the remembered distance. I kept hitting till both my hands were raw. In the evenings Geoff and I played eight ball on a fancy snooker table in the club basement. There were girls hanging about.

On one occasion I played a guy who thought himself a shark. Through a combination of sheer good luck on my part and a fluke miss on his, I won. One of the assembled girls cocked a curious eye my way. "You're not that good, are you?" she asked. For a second I felt the tug of mutual attraction, but almost immediately I sensed my scrawny self jutting out beneath my skin and maintained my silence.

That night my cousin necked with the selfsame girl by the pool. When he reported this fact, I felt a curious mix of humiliation and elation. I was back in the world—disappointed by it, certainly, but back nonetheless.

Later in the week I witnessed the moment at which my grandfather began the slow final descent towards death. He had broken his dentures, and though my mother was rushing around south Florida looking for a replacement, he seemed defeated by the sheer indignity of his predicament—stuck in Florida with no teeth. He sat in his room refusing to come out. At one stage mum insisted that we go find him and keep him company awhile, thinking we'd divert him from the bottle. When we got to his room, he was in his undershirt and boxers, sitting on the edge of the bed. He told us in a weak and rambling fashion how he'd come to meet Truman in the Oval Office. For the first time I thought of his reminiscences, "This is ancient history."

That night at dinner he lashed out at some slight in service apparent only to himself. I ran ahead as my cousin walked him back to his room, all of us having abandoned dinner in a hail of his invective, including racial epithets that rang through the place like gunshots. "Where," he demanded to know, "did all these niggers come from?" I remember feeling cowardly, running ahead pretending I was serving as an early warning for those who might take offence. "Look out," I tried to shout, "here comes my crazy old racist grandpa smashed to the gills. Would you give us a hand putting him to bed?" Nothing emerged save a strangled gargle as my cousin bravely hustled him past the mostly black staff.

My grandfather died a year or so later, his final days marked by whiskey highballs, a green garbage bag wrapped around the cushion of his favourite chair, and stacks of magazines in the midst of his exquisite library full to the brim with books that had once given him pleasure. Towards the end he took to calling me Thomas. I had a cousin of that name (Geoff's brother) and I just assumed he had mixed us up. Later I discovered from my mother that he was in fact confusing me with his dead son, my mother's brother, who had drowned (precipitated by a heart attack), aged twelve, some thirty years earlier. Having reflected a bit on this lately, I recall a photograph of my mother taken from the shoreline looking to where she sits on the green-stained stairs of our cottage. She's wearing khaki shorts and a sleeveless, floral-patterned cotton shirt. Her arms rest easy on the tops of her knees; you can see the blue veins criss-crossing the backs of her hands as they hang loose at the wrists. She's looking to the middle distance. I imagine she's watching children swim.

Until I was thirteen or so, whenever I swam, my mother insisted that she be there to "watch me." There always had to be someone there to watch me.

A little over a year after the accident, in the fall of 1975, I was deposed in an examination for discovery in a lawsuit my father had launched three days after I was run over. Where my mother fretted and fussed, dad went to court. We, the plaintiffs, were asking for $75,000 from the defendants—the truck's driver, Woodford Canning, and Somerville car and truck rentals—to redress pain and suffering and some of my father's costs. I don't remember much about the proceedings except that we settled for something in the neighbourhood of $30,000 and that the reason we did so turned on my decision not to testify further. I was standing in the kitchen when dad asked me whether I wanted to go to trial. The offer to settle was not considered sufficient either by him or by the lawyer. Dad thought we could do much better financially if we won than if we settled.

I couldn't remember why I refused him, so I dug up the record of my deposition, taken September 8, 1975, high up in a downtown office tower. Before being called in I remember noticing a man who looked like a bowling ball glancing over at me, then looking away. I assumed this was the guy who ran over me. I imagined he thought he should have finished the job. As I testified, a man at one end of the table spoke into what looked like one of those oxygen masks that are supposed to drop out of the ceiling of an airplane if anything goes wrong during the flight.

My lawyer's name is O'Brien and the defendant's lawyer is Davison:

Mr. O'Brien: Are you through with the injuries, Mr. Davison?
Mr. Davison: I think I am. Why?
Mr. O'Brien: There is a scar that is quite unsightly on the stomach.
Mr. Davison : Yes, I was going to ask him about that. Does the scar show, Doug, when you wear a bathing suit?
A: Yes.

BY MR. DAVISON
Q: Speaking only about the scar, does it bother you physically? Is there pain or tingling or anything like that?
A: It itches.
Q: How do you feel about the scar?
A: Well, I don't know. I try not to let it bother me.

Q: Maybe I had better have a look at it, if you don't mind.

Mr. O'Brien: I had some pictures taken.

Mr. Davison: Can I just see how it looks now? [At this point I must have lifted my shirt and stood with my bare midriff in plain view.] It looks to me as though there's more than one. Those are . . . I take it the other marks are from this injury and the tubes and so on?

Mr. O'Brien: Yes. I think they had removed an abscess on a couple of them.

BY MR. DAVISON

Q: Does it go down below your belt?

A: There is another one down here, just over here.

Q: What is it? I see. Is that the lowest one?

A: Yes

Q: How far does the vertical one go?

A: That's it right there.

Q: So it is about six to eight inches long, depending on whether you are breathing in or out?

A: Yes.

Q: And it is accompanied by four other smaller scars?

A: Right.

Q: Three of them appear to be circular and another one is . . .

A: Oblong.

Q: Oblong, and they are all dark substantially in colour. Have you asked the doctor about the scars? Have you asked about them, as to whether or not they are going to change in colour or any thing like that?

A: Yes.

Q: What did he say?

A: The thing about the way I heal is, I heal . . . I don't remember the exact medical term for it, but usually most scars kind of heal in, whereas mine kind of stay out.

Mr. O'Brien: Keloid.

A: And they will whiten eventually.

BY MR. DAVISON

Q: Have you seen a plastic surgeon with relation to the scars?

A: They don't bother me that much.

Q: Pardon?

A: They don't bother me that much.

Q: The scrapes and other things we talked about didn't leave any scarring, I take it?

A: No. It's gone *okay*. No.

When my lawyerly wife, the hard-driving, stay-up-twenty-four-hours deal-closing fiend, read this, she turned to me in bed and said, "That's horrible. How could your lawyer let them do that to you?" I guess I know now why I insisted on settling the suit. And though I can't remember exactly, there's something in that word "okay" that tells me how I must have been feeling. "It's gone *okay*." In other words, "What I mean to say is, I'm gone. I'm scrawny and I'm gone, you dick. Girls generally don't like scrawny guys, which is mostly everything I think about, so yeah, actually, now that you mention it, it does bother me."

But no, I don't really remember what I thought. I do remember the defendant's lawyer, Mr. Davison, had a chunky gold ring on his middle finger and hairy knuckles.

I thought the ring was garish and that his hands were just plain unattractive. Afterwards, Dad and I walked to his car. I asked how he thought things had gone. Dad paused a moment, his mouth working itself into the vaguely wry expression I'd seen a zillion times. "I thought things went rather well except when they asked you what you thought you might want to *be* . . ."

"Yeah yeah," I interjected. "I should have said I wanted to be a pro hockey player or something."

"Or even better," said my father, knowing what he'd just seen and hoping to reduce the impact by making light of it, "a bodybuilder."

I couldn't wait to get to school to tell someone my dad's joke.

Where my father's sense of humour was dry as dust, mum's was somewhat more . . . liquidy. At Christmastime for several years running my mother asked a guy named Raymond Archer to come round and help decorate the Christmas tree. Raymond was floridly gay, given to extravagant gestures and expressions over just about everything. Things were "fabulous" or "crazy" or "exquisite." Raymond was a talented painter and designer who'd done wonderful *trompe l'oeil* decorations on a variety of wood surfaces throughout our house. He was sufficiently gifted that even in my philistine fifteen-year-old state I knew he was doing something worthy of respect.

The afternoon I remember particularly would have occurred in early December 1975. I had arrived home from school to discover mum and Raymond decorating the tree. I plunked down on the couch, ostensibly to read but really to listen to the entirely entertaining byplay between the two yuletide artistes. (My mother loved to patronize smart gay men of the decorator/florist class. The ones she liked were outrageously funny, gossipy and tender; in other words the reverse of most of the heterosexual men who peopled the class from which mother and I sprang. And I was attracted to them for the same reasons as my mum.) My book was *Bert Fegg's Nasty Book for Boys and Girls*, a brilliant parody of British juvenile literature by Pythons Michael Palin and Terry Jones. Instead of listening, I quickly found myself snorting and chuckling at the brilliant perversity of it all.

Raymond interrupted his half of the gin-soaked colloquy to ask, "What, pray tell, are you reading?"

I averred that I was reading *Bert Fegg's Nasty Book for Boys and Girls*, specifically a musical play titled "Aladdin and His Terrible Problem" whose two lead characters were named Pisso (an alcoholic dog) and Depravo (a rat friend of Pisso's).

The title alone delighted Raymond and he declared with a swishy flourish, "You must sing it for us at once."

So I did. It's impossible in print to get at the essence of this, since the weight of its hilarity was borne in the moment. But for the sake of trying, imagine my only slightly post-pubescent voice producing the following song, complete with appropriate estuary British inflection:

Depravo (sings):
I'm Depravo Depravo the Rat
As filthy a creature as can be
I'm vicious and ill tempered,
I make everybody jump,
I cheat and lie and swindle,
And smell like a rubbish dump.

I haven't a heart of gold,
I've no redeeming feature
I'm Depravo the Rat
A truly filthy creature
Chorus:
He's Depravo . . . Depravo the Rat
The biggest health hazard in Peking
Depravo:
I like being very rude
Eating half digested food
And seeing ladies in the nude...

I remember my mother and Raymond collapsing to their knees at this, and me thinking I might just be the funniest guy in Creation.

The following summer I went to the Olympics in Montreal. I was staying with the Scotts, assigned to my cousin Geoff and two of his chums from Bishop's College School in Lennoxville. We were all sixteen, and we were all from approximately the same social and economic station. One major difference, however: they had bodies like Michelangelo's *David* and I did not. I hung listlessly around the local pub, still scrawny from the accident, while my cousin and his cronies purred like Lamborghinis, seducing the local talent. Getting noticed, I figured, would require an act of outlandish eccentricity. *De l'audace, encore de l'audace, toujours de l'audace*. Though I likely wouldn't have known what Danton's dictum meant, I was a certain, if unconscious, practitioner of its counsel.

Because the boys had patronage jobs at the Olympic drug-testing facilities for equestrian events and I did not, they had money and I did not. Pride may have prevented me from borrowing coin sufficient to fund an evening's worth of beer; I don't remember. Still, I had a plan. As the boys made their way to the dance floor or elsewhere, I would slip around and test the temperature of abandoned draft beers with my finger. The warmer the draft, the better—it meant that its imbiber had probably gone out to the parking lot, there to spoon a couple of hours away, and was less likely to miss the beer when he got back, foggy-eyed.

Down the hatch!

Geoff was going with Toni Shaw, a bosomy girl with a face as open as any window in spring. When told of my beery exploits, she looked at me with an expression I'd like to think was half-puzzled, half-intrigued. Not that it mattered—I was pissed and, for the moment, content, the anxiety of sexual inferiority washed away on a warm tide.

When I returned to high school that fall, I continued to drink. This wasn't a good idea. My marks stunk. I was mouthy and unrepentant. My life seemed unhinged. On her deathbed my mother remembered me after the accident as a kid who just didn't give a damn. "You wanted something else, but you didn't know what, and no one could tell you anything. You didn't want to know."

When I think of it now, I want to rush back and reassure myself that everything I felt was okay. "Let's face it," I'd say, "life sucks. The only difference between you and these other rubes is that at least you know it."

At Christmas in Grade 12 my marks bottomed out. Fifty-six percent. My mother looked defeated. My father didn't speak of it.

Sometime after Christmas, I started getting wicked pains in my belly. I remember spending afternoons and early evenings during the late winter and early spring of 1977 curled up in a fetal position on my bed, the pain a distant though audible echo dulled only by several hits from my mother's bottle of 222s. I think I might have been hooked on the stuff. I was wickedly constipated, a side effect of the codeine. Of course I didn't utter a word to anyone, inventing for my own relief a phony context for this disaster waiting to happen. To my mind I was a stoic braving the agony so as not to be a burden. In fact, I was dead scared. The episodes of pain became more frequent. One night before a math test I was up till four a.m. rolling around in bed, wishing away the pain.

On April 30, 1977, my parents went out to dinner. Normally this was a treat since it afforded me a chance to watch TV, a pastime banned during the week. Shortly after they left, however, the pain hit with a vengeance. I went to the medicine chest and gobbled down several 222s. No good. I wandered around the house—no, I crawled, rolled and clawed at the carpet, looking for any measure of relief. There was none. When my parents got home, my mother took one look at me and quickly called Clint Stephens at home. Her voice had an anxious, pleading quality that embarrassed me.

Stephens found his way to the house in a matter of minutes. The pain felt as though something was pushing hard from the inside, trying to get out. Dad had taken a few drinks and was more sorrowful than comforting. There was about him the pungent odor of whiskey. The doctor palpated my belly in his reassuring way. Nausea and pain swept over me, and I fell to my knees and puked into a trash bin lined with a brown paper bag. The vomit dripped between the liner and the tin as I stared at the illustration on the outside of the basket, some nineteenth-century scene of hounds and huntsmen chasing their prey.

I was admitted to Sick Kids' hospital that night—at seventeen, the oldest kid in the place. Since my wrecked duodenum had recovered, it was decided that the jejunostomy that had linked my stomach directly to my bowel would be undone. The pain was put down to a bowel obstruction, though no evidence was found to support this diagnosis. The "degastrojejunostomy" was a precaution against ulcers later in life.

I came to in a dark recovery room. My mother was by the bed. She read me a report from the *Toronto Sun* recounting the Football Association Cup soccer match pitting Manchester United against Liverpool. Mum read it with every ounce of passion and feeling she could muster for a story about which she cared not a whit. Imagine my mother's emphatic, theatrical voice, full of musical emphasis, crucial words drawn out, now legato, now diminuendo, traipsing across the lead: "Liver-pooool's *dream* of adding the English Football Association Cup to its league soccer TITLE was *shattered* yesterday by a 2–1 loss to Manchester United in the cup final at Wembley."

I recovered from the operation quickly and without complication, and was discharged on May 14. I was home for a week. I remember going to Stephens's office in the yellowy grey Medical Arts Building on St. George Street and having a surgically implanted feeding tube yanked from my stomach. The next morning I woke up with a pain so intense I asked immediately to go to the hospital. (Note the contrast between this response and the phony heroics of previous weeks.) The pain seemed to come from somewhere down very deep inside me and to radiate through my trunk. It was steady and certain, offering no release at all.

As mum drove me down to the hospital, the agony was relentless, unremitting. The reasonable response to pain—"I'm sick, I have to ride this out"—seemed wholly inadequate. It pushed me beyond the merely circumstantial and into the realm of moral culpability. This can't just be happening to me; *somebody* must be at fault. What have I done to deserve this? I felt as though I were receding inside myself, seeking someplace to hide from the pain.

Following my readmission I was moved from my bed on the ward down to the X-ray department. They wanted to monitor the progress of a barium dose through my digestive tract to see if another blockage was fomenting all this misery. The hospital records describing the course of that examination make only tangential reference to the acute nature of my pain. "The exam was limited because of the extreme restlessness of the patient." The *Oxford English Dictionary* defines "restless" as follows: "deprived of rest; finding no rest; *esp.* uneasy in mind or spirit." Language is always inadequate on these occasions.

I was rolled back and forth on the ice-cold examining table as a variety of nurses and technicians tugged me around to get a better picture. I produced noises I'd never heard before. I felt myself heave under the weight of a pressure so immense and grotesque I had no sense of its dimensions. I was stripped of sentiment. For relief I would have killed anyone in that room, slit their throats and watched them die like dogs at my feet.

Later, returned to the ward, I was so weary that I could feel the effort required to open my eyes. It was like holding up a barbell with both arms extended straight out from my chest. If I let go, my eyelids came crashing down like heavy blinds suddenly untethered.

I was wheeled along by a nurse who'd been responsible for babysitting me in earlier times. Her name was Liz McMaster, a jokey, needling sort. She was at it again now, trying to buoy me up with some patter or other. I remember thinking that she ought to just shut up. I kept my face blank, partly because I was so exhausted and partly because I thought it might torture her. Her expression changed to one of alarm and concern. "Jesus," she muttered, "you really are sick."

From there, I remember fragments of sight and sound, with little co-ordination between the two. I heard Stephens order me a dose of Demerol. The next thing, my eyes opened on several doctors and nurses, gloved and gowned, their faces half covered with surgical masks.

Under the entry headed "state of patient on arrival in o.r." someone has written the word "apprehensive." In fact, I had looked around the room and, as I felt no immediate pain (mostly, I suppose, thanks to the Demerol), expressed first my confusion, then my displeasure. *Why would you wake me up only to put me back to sleep? Couldn't we all just take a minute and think about this?* I started to protest further when I caught Dr. Stephens's ice blue eyes, which betrayed a certain amusement. He said something reassuring, and moments later I felt the rush of unconsciousness whirling all around me.

Then something really weird happened. Having been anaesthetized several times, I knew I was on the brink of unconsciousness when I heard a sound not unlike the Doppler effect produced by a passing race car; as the car passes, the sound diminishes. And so it was with my diminishing consciousness as the anaesthetic was applied. This time I heard the sound allright, even felt some part of my conscious mind slip away, and yet I didn't go under. For the first few minutes of the operation I actually heard the goings-on inside the operating theatre. I heard them tape my eyes shut, heard them prepare my midsection with orange disinfectant. Because I had no way of communicating my discomfort at being aware of all this, I felt a thoroughly impotent panic rush through me. Soon, however, I realized there was absolutely nothing to be done and I actually began to enjoy the proceedings. It was a bit like listening to a radio play in which you're the plot.

In the course of three weeks I'd been subjected to two laparotomies. On this occasion the intent was purely exploratory. The doctors had no idea what was wrong, so they opened me up like a car to look under the hood. The report describing the surgery reveals a straightforward procedure that ultimately resulted in a relatively unproblematic diagnosis: "the head of the pancreas was somewhat enlarged and firm . . . an amylase taken just while the operation started, from the blood, showed a serum amylase of over 2000 units." All of which pointed to acute pancreatitis as the culprit. Acute pancreatitis is a condition of the pancreas wherein that little-known organ, tucked away deep inside the abdominal cavity and responsible for producing insulin and amylase, a digestive enzyme, betrays its cause and runs roughshod over the body. During the attack the organ, which overflows with nerve endings, in essence digests itself, causing severe pain. It is generally conceded to be among the most painful conditions of the body.

(Only one item in the report left my grown-up self feeling cold. The surgeons had run a catheter through my digestive system. "There was no obstruction, however on putting the catheter in the duodenum a peculiar, yellowy, mucousy liquid was obtained." It is particularly disturbing to read that doctors, while looking at a place you will never see, discovered something even they found "peculiar." Which is, according to the OED, "singular, strange, odd or queer." This is *not* good.)

The report insists that at the conclusion of the procedure I was "feeling well." In fact, I felt godawful, and the running tally of Demerol shots supports this. Reading the nursing assessments, I'm surprised by the degree to which my curiosity about my condition disturbed, intrigued or at least puzzled my caregivers. "[Patient is]... very alert, responsive, intelligent and pleasant. No sign of depression but concerned over long term effects of surgery... asking many questions re sedation, i.e. how often; when next—what will it be—Demerol?... seems overly concerned with sedation demanding to know what type it is, says that it works better psychologically if you know what it is... continues to be interested plus, plus, plus in sedation... asking many questions re pain, and sedation not working ... talking plus, plus, plus about illness, medications, (sedation etc.) and what the next few weeks will be like. Continues to be very interested in his own illness and treatment—knows just when he can have sedation asks for k basin directly after sedation 'in case he gets nauseous.'" I understand that these nurses needed to treat me in a certain way, like a malfunctioning toaster, in order to keep their professional distance, but I am still surprised to discover that the talking toaster was such a revelation.

In point of fact there was quite a lot that I didn't feel I needed to share with the nurses. Ten days or so after the surgery I was still receiving doses of Demerol on demand to keep me out of pain's way. One shot struck me as not quite as necessary as the ones that preceded it. It was given in the meaty part of the thigh and, as always, the warming effect seemed to spread right through me, slowly at first, then rapidly and inexorably, like tidal waters washing over a strand. But whereas that tide had previously resulted in a restored a sense of equilibrium, this time it not only defeated the pain handily, but kept on going all the way to Moscow.

I felt suddenly very light, like I was drifting just above the bed, held aloft by a cushion of pleasure. I was, in a word, baked. There was a hockey game playing on a television high up in one corner of the room. It was the final game in the Avco Cup series, the short-lived World Hockey Association's equivalent to the Stanley Cup, named for a Winnipeg-based trust company. Now, I was an avid, even fanatical, sports fan. And the Avco Cup would, even under normal circumstances, have garnered a large share of my attention, as it pitted the Winnipeg Jets and the still impressive Bobby Hull against the Quebec Nordiques. But the degree to which this particular game riveted, fascinated and enthralled me was disproportionate to my interest in hockey (or should I say, to any sober man's interest in just about anything). At one stage the players actually seemed to leave the screen and skate a swirling, ghostly pattern around me. And so it went—the players drifting around me, then returning to the screen and out again.

I must have fallen asleep because, when I came to, the room was black and a nurse was standing by the bed holding my wrist. "What happened to the hockey players?" I heard myself ask. I wanted them back. I asked for another shot.

Though there's no record of my having been in any way addicted to Demerol, I'm almost certain that the final game of the 1976/77 WHA season marked my last purely recreational encounter with that drug.

It was a slow recovery this time. I seemed to drift in and out of focus even more than I had during my much lengthier stay after the accident. I have one very strong recollection, however. A teacher from my school came to see me, Jock Armitage, for whom I had the greatest affection. It was an odd pairing, really. Armitage was the senior maths instructor, a subject for which I demonstrated little or no aptitude. But he had another interest, which most of the other masters didn't share: fellowship. Among his duties he ran the book room, a glorified cupboard from which he sold books and supplies. At the noon hour I would go there, sit down with my sandwich, drink and fruit cup, and chat. Whatever the subject, he entered the conversation with good will. He didn't seem to feel the need to prove in the first five or six seconds that he was smarter than me, that he was credentialled or otherwise authorized. I cherish the memory of those conversations now, though I barely remember what they were about, only that I always felt better for having them.

Mr. Armitage came to the hospital and we started to talk just as we had before. Although I was lying there with tubes sticking out of most orifices, he had the innate ability to make the conversation flow. He told me that in my absence I had been elected head of house. I knew he had rigged it for me, and I knew that at least one other had to have been disappointed. I was at the same moment discomfited and elated. I got the prize because I was sick, because he felt sorry for me. But I still won the prize, and it made me want to be well.

Years later, when he retired from St. George's, Jock Armitage sent me his own house tie in the mail.

The following spring was, by the standards of personal mythology, among my finest seasons. I was appointed a prefect at Christmas. I had a girlfriend. I won the school's most prestigious athletic award in recognition of my "courage" and received a standing ovation from my schoolmates and their parents at the awards ceremony. As I walked to the front of the room to receive the plaque, I kept my head down. Was it humility or shame? I can't quite remember.

That spring one of my classmates, Ian Lomax, went into the hospital. He had leukemia. Tall and lean, Lomax was a superbly intuitive athlete with a dry sense of humour. He was very smart. His best friend was Glen Ollers, a Swede with a similar frame and sensibility. The previous winter I had watched Ian, already suffering the ravaging effects of the disease, put on the purest display of frantic athleticism I've ever seen. His stamina was handicapped, but he was still good for short bursts off the bench. The precise circumstances of the basketball game are lost to me, but I remember the coach calling him to go in and Ian springing like a steel coil to the task. He played five, maybe six minutes, and he was everywhere, especially on defence, blocking shots, leaping to intercept passes, crouching low to cover his man, his face a mask of pure aggression. The opposing players looked as though they were seeing something for the first time, a quality both beautiful and horrible to behold. At one stage Ian tied the ball up for a jump. Just as the whistle sounded, he tore the ball from the opponent's hands and for a moment there was a wolfish ardour about him, as though he might devour the ball and his opponent too, if it came to that. After he came off, the sweat was pouring off him, his head and body draped in towels.

One Saturday afternoon the following spring, Ollers organized us to go visit Ian at St. Joseph's Hospital. His room was dimly lit. Jesus writhed on a cross over his bed.

We stood in the room and watched him die a little. His lips were parched. Every so often he asked for water. Periodically his body arched with a pain that, like an angry surf, left a little less of him each time it waned. We lasted about forty minutes. Glen was agitated on the drive home, insisting that we needed to tell our classmates what was really going on at the hospital.

Ian died a couple of weeks later. That night our entire year gathered at a classmate's house. Nobody knew how to behave, so everybody got drunk. I felt noble and righteous facing death half-cut.

PANIC

To confront with forgiveness and compassion the terrifying singularity of my own person.

—JOHN CHEEVER

THE IMMEDIATE REPERCUSSIONS of my first bout with pancreatitis were relatively minor. I was moved onto a low-fat diet, something that was quite exotic in the late seventies. My mother was forever trooping off to some far-flung wholesale specialty shop or, even more improbable, ordering nutritional supplements through the mail. Low-fat brownies, sherbets, dried low-fat bean soup, skim milk cheese: these were the staples of my diet.

A Texas football coach, forced to change his eating habits, was asked the contents of his new diet. "Ah cawl it the spit-it-out diet," he drawled. "If it taystes good, spit it out."

This was hardly a problem for me, as nothing tasted of anything. My mother was relentless and, from my adolescent perspective, hysterical regarding my dietary intake. Initially, fear of her wrath and an excess of supervision kept me from straying. But that passed, and I found myself sneaking over to Senior's restaurant on Yonge Street just south of St. Clair, a dark, meaty establishment stinking of grilled fat, to down a steak or a smoked-meat sandwich. I didn't spit it out. And as I lost the discipline of her instruction, the very idea of curtailing my diet fell away. I couldn't wait to wiggle free of my mother's clutches.

In early September, 1978, with mum behind the wheel, we raced along the 401 in her Volkswagen towards Kingston, and Queen's University. I'd never set eyes on the place. All I knew was that it was 150 miles east of Toronto and that, besides the odd weekend and holidays (I was *seeking* independence, I wasn't independent per se), I would be left to my own devices. If there was a theme that rode right through my years as an undergraduate, that was it. Left to my own devices, I behaved with reckless disregard for my own health and best interests. On that first day I remember walking across the quad among the various prison block residences, amidst the mad, bad behaviour of orientation or "frosh" week, and turning several times to shoo my mother away until she finally stood staring after me, her hand splayed on the hood of the car.

I continued to drink at an accelerating pace. I chased girls and sought out a relentless social schedule, with mixed results. I failed to take hold of my studies, the usual mixed bag of first-year humanities courses—philosophy, English, history and politics—with any constancy, but for the first couple of years I got by with a gentleman's B (minus). I struggled with my freedom to an unhealthy degree precisely because I put far too much faith in its rewards.

During my first term I handed in a short essay on *Pride and Prejudice*, the first writing of my university career. As it happened, the professor, a shy, stuttering mess of a woman, decided to read my piece to the assembled as an example of what was required of first-year English essays. (I did not attend as I was profoundly hung over.) After this was reported to me, I attended exactly one more class that year, during which a buxom member of the Queen's field hockey team asked me if I would help her with her studies. I never saw her again either. I didn't hand in the rest of my papers till the day after the marks were due. The professor looked utterly incredulous as I shoved a mitt full of incoherent ramblings at her. I could go into the twisted rationalizations and deep underlying insecurities that led to this behaviour, but I'm guessing you're a bright person and can work it out for yourself. Oh, and if you do figure it out, let me know.

For most of my first year I was in a sort of ongoing social panic, whether I was studying, conversing, drinking or dancing. I held in my mind some platonic form of whatever it was that I was doing to remind me that somewhere there was something better and I better go find it. I was, in short, a jerk.

I wasn't so much a social climber as a social paranoid. Whereas every death diminished John Donne because he was involved in mankind, every social gathering to which I was not invited diminished me because I was so monumentally self-involved. Anxiety was a constant companion. By my third year at Queen's this skittishness had evolved into episodic panic attacks.

That fall I was dating a woman, Margot, for whom I had a considerable sexual appetite. Margot was an athlete, a former national-level freestyle skier with a pragmatic turn of mind. What she was doing with me is still a puzzle. She had a fabulous room that took up the entire third floor of a capacious house near campus. Heaven on earth. I travelled there at all hours, freezing cold, slipping between the sheets and feeling her warmth flow directly to my groin. My roommates that year sent me a birthday card that read, "From the boys at 198 Division Street—Remember us? The guys you *live* with." I laughed uncomfortably at this. I even felt guilty enough that I dragged Margot back to my filthy room now and again thereafter, to fuck and sleep fitfully on a ratty single bed.

One night early in the new year of 1981 we had smoked several spliffs and were in the midst of a post-coital snuggle when suddenly I couldn't catch my breath. It felt as though my heart had stopped. I sat up straight and said that I was about to die. Margot took the reasonable course, suggesting that I was having a paranoid response to the dope. What she failed to realize was that I was nuts from top to bottom, stoned turtles all the way down. The idea that my heart might stop because I was impaired was trumped by the idea that it might stop because six years earlier it almost had.

I did the only thing I thought might save my life. Abandoning the skeptical Margot, I ran naked, in sub-zero temperatures, to a house next door full of women I knew and admired, and banged on their door. At three in the morning. Luckily, I suppose, one of Margot's roommates dragged me off the porch before I managed to demand rescue from the neighbours. Then he and Margot drove me to the hospital.

In Emergency, I explained my medical history to a doctor. It was the beginning of a ten-year cycle, all following pretty much the same script. After the explanation came the examination. Due to the severity of my previous illnesses this was probably a good deal more exhaustive than physicals afforded your run-of-the-mill panic artist. Blood tests for sure, and on the odd occasion an X-ray or ultrasound. Then, after an hour or so, the doctor would reappear, always with a slightly quizzical look, often fidgeting with the test results that stared up from one of those metallic medical clipboards.

"The tests are negative. We're pretty sure it's not your liver or your pancreas. You haven't been under any undue stress or strain of late, have you?"

"Uh, not really, not that I'm aware of."

The doctor would then suggest I might want to seek some counselling on stress management. In retrospect, this would probably have been a good idea. (Oh, screw it, I know I'm supposed to think that, but the truth is I wouldn't trade any of my conduct since. There was a wildness and ferocity about me that makes for great fodder.) Thinking of it, I see the continuities and discontinuities between life now and life then, and I always come back to mum: "You wanted something else, but you didn't know what and no one could tell you anything. You were at loose ends." I saw myself as having two speeds with which to proceed through life. Let's call them comatose and caterwauling.

Later that year a bunch of friends and I piled into Margot's station wagon and drove to Toronto. We'd been invited to a party thrown by one of Canada's richest men to celebrate his son's twenty-first birthday. For me it was proof positive that the super rich *are* different. I remember a lot of balloons floating in a sub-lit aqua pool that made everything seem hyper-festive. I decided it was vulgar and would forever seem vulgar unless at some point in the future I could afford to throw a party with that many balloons, and then it would seem to be among the best ideas I'd ever had. I drank vats of champagne and chatted up the twenty-one-year-old's much younger sister. At the end of the evening I staggered towards the DJ and asked if he could play a song by the Clash entitled "The Sound of the Sinners," a swinging gospel number from *Sandinista!* My drunken vocal chords produced "Kooyoo . . . lay de shlounnd . . . e shlinners? . . . Iss byee te lasch." Looking back, I suppose I must have been *very* drunk, because I was surprised, offended even, at my inability to get this sentence out in anything remotely resembling English. "Hey," I thought deep in the bowels of my mind, "who's been fucking around with my brain." I don't know how the DJ figured it out, but the platter in question was soon spinning away.

The song, as I say, is rousing, and in a moment everyone was up pole-hopping about. I felt myself swaying dangerously one way and then the other, but like a weeble I wobbled yet never quite fell down.

The next morning (having returned to Margot's parents' north Toronto house—how, I can't remember) I was awoken by a tremendous pressure in my lower abdomen. I was still drunk and, being that way, didn't fully realize the implications. I had slept on a couch but had no idea how I got there. As I stood, I found I was holding my right hand perpendicular to my face, in the manner of half a Hindu greeting. It seemed I needed a navigational aid, like the horizon gauge on a plane's control panel, to keep me on a steady path to the washroom. For reasons that remain mysterious to me, I decided instead to pee over the banister and down the back stairs. In a flash Margot was standing beside me on the landing, asking me what the hell I was doing. I heard two braided sounds: Margot's plaintive voice and howls of laughter from two friends who were sitting in the kitchen into which a steady stream of urine was flowing. National Lampoon once put out an album of comedy bits titled *that's not funny, that's sick*. I now know exactly on which side of the line my behaviour fell. At the time my judgement was less certain.

Margot packed me into the rear of her station wagon for the trip back to Kingston with newspapers spread out beneath me, as if I were a yet-to-be-housebroken dog. I was humiliated, vilified even, by those who'd found my antics amusing. (Not too long thereafter Margot decided, after two years of moi, to throw her lot in with a stable chartered accountant named, I kid you not, Roland Nimmo. They're still married, have innumerable children and from all accounts are incredibly happy.) The boy-man's loose ends were flailing in his wake like tether straps bouncing on the highway behind a flatbed truck.

By my fifth and final year at Queen's ("fifth year" being something of a joke among undergraduates, a backwater for the dim and the disorganized), I hung around the humanities building like a monk around the cloister. Though comically disorganized, I was finally engaged by my studies, even picking up the odd A in philosophy courses that required only essays for assessment. Exams or tests of any kind were a disaster. I was trying desperately to raise my abysmal academic standing so that I might find my way to graduate school, as I had no other prospect and no thought of a prospect.

I can see now that my performance wasn't as dismal as I imagined at the time. In addition to my studies I was organizing, through the auspices of Frontier College, a national charitable institution for basic adult education, fellow students to teach prison inmates to read. (Kingston, a good, grey limestone town harkening back to its vedy, vedy British roots, has a weird high/low quality what with a university, six or so prisons, a military college and an inordinate number of institutions of every stripe.) I was attracted to Frontier College because it combined a tradition of radicalism—Norman Bethune was among its teaching alumni—with establishment credentials. Most importantly, it was a safe haven to work through my limousine liberal misgivings about entitlement.

Keeping a foot in every camp was my game. My closest friends at Queen's referred to me as the chameleon. I took this as a compliment, though I suspect it wasn't offered as one. As for my performance in philosophy, I was always of the view that any prof who gave me a decent grade couldn't see that I was pulling the wool over his or her eyes. Beneath my baroque rationalizations, my taste in philosophical reasoning was at best suspect. I liked the Continentals: Nietzsche and his postmodern heirs Foucault, Derrida, Feyerabend, Rorty and Stanley Fish. I was attracted to the idea that truth is relative to context. This let me off the hook. No need to knock yourself silly trying to figure things out. If everything's relative, any answer, so long as it's sufficiently articulate, is as good as any other. In my last year I received an A in moral philosophy. I did so on the basis of an essay arguing against moral relativism in a critique of a book called *After Virtue* by Alistair MacIntyre. I knew the professor, a rabid rationalist, would ken to my arguments. And so it went. If I succeded, it was because the professor was a fool; if I failed, it was because I hadn't "tried."

This insanely schizoid assessment of my own abilities coloured my entire academic career.

In October 1982, I spent an evening at the grad pub drinking beer and watching the Milwaukee Brewers and the St. Louis Cardinals playing for the World Series. I was in the company of two fellow humanities students—Adam, a graduate student in philosophy, and Michael, a fourth-year English student. I had some money down on Milwaukee, enough that I imagined I couldn't afford to lose it. As Milwaukee faltered, I began to see my money slipping away. However, there was something more sinister taking hold of me. It was as if for the first time I sensed the sheer futility of my situation. Adam and Mike were like channel buoys pointing the way to my failings. Adam was disciplined and perseverant. Mike was incandescent—a brilliantly intuitive thinker with both intellectual and artistic gifts. I was neither.

The game ended and we decided to go back to work. We were a bit in our cups, but not so much that the idea of work seemed absurd. We paused in the lobby to get cups of coffee. I slotted in the thirty-five cents and waited as the machine began its usual round of whirs and burps on its way to dropping a cup. Only this time the cup didn't drop. The coffee started to flow out of the machine, splattering and hissing into the space where the cup was meant to be. That machine, I thought, is truly fucked. I started to bemoan my fate, loudly. To my mind I was kidding, but there was something in Mike's expression that suggested he thought otherwise. I started hitting the machine and saying something like, "Can you *believe* it"—smacking the machine for emphasis, timing my strikes to punctuate the latter syllable of the word "believe." On the third strike it felt as though a light bulb had exploded at the centre of my brain. I ran across the lobby, falling and twisting, repeating rapid fire the words "fuck me, fuck me, fuck me, fuck me." I was beginning to wonder whether I was dramatizing my condition when I looked down and saw vivid crimson splashed across my yellow sweater. "Jesus," I heard Adam say.

I looked up and saw him take off like a shot. Then I looked at my wrist. There was what looked to be an enormous flap of skin leaking blood. It didn't seem to be squirting out, which I found reassuring. I went into a bathroom and ran some cold water onto the gash. I wrapped the wrist in paper towels and held my hand over my head as though holding up the pole inside a collapsing tent. In the meantime Mike had called a cab. While we waited, I asked Mike what had happened to Adam. "I think he ran to the hospital." I remember thinking that Adam was in good enough shape to do it.

At the hospital, a nurse appeared and I had to actively resist saying, "Here, fix this." She started to reach up for my hand and I pulled away. "I have to look at it," she said impatiently, and began to peel off the sticky layers of paper towel. I looked away. Her first clinical comment was, "Oh, shit."

I replied, "Hey, how bad can it be? Didn't they teach you at nursing school to say something reassuring, like 'Don't worry, you'll live?'"

Mike looked hard at me as the nurse led me towards a curtained-off bay. "Doug, shut up. Shut the fuck up."

There was another bed on my left, occupied by a man shackled with a handcuff to the rail. My right arm, draped in green towels, was extended at a ninety-degree angle from my body.

"What the fuck happened to you?" he growled.

I struggled to find an appropriately hard-nosed response. "I uh I um aah punched out a coffee machine." Here I paused and added for emphasis, "*man*." I turned my head away before my interlocutor had a chance to respond.

Not another word passed between us.

The doctors and nurses proceeded to patch me up as best they could and told me to turn up for surgery the next day to repair the nerve damage. Mike had stuck around and Adam had reappeared. I was given some Percodan to get me through. As we all lived within a couple of blocks of each other in downtown Kingston, we decided to share a cab, which moved at a snail's pace along the deserted streets. We eyeballed each other in silence; something was very wrong with our driver. Before we could speak up, the cabbie turned to us. "Do you fellas mind if I pull over a second?" He swung onto one of the side streets heading down to Lake Ontario, but instead of pulling over he simply let the cab coast into a parked car. The cab jerked to a halt and our heads bobbed simultaneously. The cabbie looked at us balefully. "Uh sorry, I just need a minute." We slid out of the car, leaving our drunk driver to mumble about us skipping out on the fare.

It was very late. I was very stoned on Percodan. As we walked along, the three of us started to cackle like crows.

The next morning I called my father, trying to disguise my voice with a cloak of *savoir faire*. That lasted about five seconds. Dad dressed me down, but there wasn't much to be done. I was scheduled for surgery in a couple of hours.

Those moments leading up to surgery are desperate in the way of any circumstance where all semblance of self-control has been stripped away. There you are, draped in a green sheet. Your extremities are freezing. Nurses and the odd doctor stare at you, their faces hidden by surgical masks. In my case I looked around the theatre for some reassurance, and fixed on a particularly attractive set of blue eyes. "As these may be my final few moments on this earth, I'd like to give you my phone number. It's 544-3602."

"Try to calm down," the eyes responded, "everything's going to be fine. Please count back from 100."

I heard a voice on the intercom asking the surgeon to call a Dr. Harrison at Sunnybrook Hospital regarding Douglas Bell. *Urgent.*

"Hey," said the surgeon, "I know that guy." He then turned to me and, sounding more annoyed than impressed, asked, "So, who do you know?"

I interrupted my countdown to respond weakly, "My dad . . . he . . . hospital head guy . . ."

As I drifted off on a pentothal cloud, I heard, "What'd he say?"

"I dunno. Let's just get on with it."

As it turned out, despite my father's well-intentioned efforts from afar, the surgery didn't do much good. I had to wear a cast for two months and suffered terrific nerve pain throughout the period of recovery. When the cast was removed, I had no measurable improvement in sensation in my hand and was directed to the department of occupational therapy at Sunnybrook Hospital. An earnest therapist suggested that the best way to improve the feeling in the tips of my fingers would be to pour a bunch of metal nuts and bolts into a coffee can along with a dried-soup mix, then repeatedly reach in and try to discern the objects from amongst the finer-grained particles. I did this until I realized that I had just spent the better part of an hour fishing around in soup mix trying to pull out the odd nut or bolt. The therapist suggested I could take the can and practise at home. To this day a coffee can full of soup mix, nuts and bolts sits untended in my basement.

In the late spring of 1983, I headed off to Calgary under the auspices of Frontier College to join a rail gang as a labourer teacher. (The job is exactly as the title would suggest: you work as a labourer on the gang and teach in your off-hours.) A certain pall came over my mother as I prepared to make my way west. I'd just finished mangling my hand, and the accompanying scar looked exactly as if I'd tried to off myself. It was clear to her that her only son was off to work with greasy roughnecks with whom he had little affinity, at a job for which he had little inclination, at a time when he looked as though he'd recently lost his mind. I wouldn't necessarily have disagreed, but at twenty-three, all evidence to the contrary, the world still seemed a place designed to accommodate the ideal ambitions of youth.

And so, one morning I headed for the airport, sporting an enormous blue knapsack with shiny new steel-toed Greb boots hanging by their laces off the back.

I managed the summer all right. Oh, there were the usual wacky misadventures. I got a nickname (Jughead, something about having gone to college and the word *jug* rhyming with Doug). I split my pants (totally inappropriate blinding white corduroy trousers) down the ass the first day. I partook, or rather failed to partake, in bar fights (for the most part hiding under chairs, respecting the advice of a Newfoundlander who told me earnestly, "Jughead, don't let 'em touch youze cause if dey can touch youze dey can probably kill youze"). In Banff, I took a magic mushroom and reported straight-facedly that it had no effect, to which my companion retorted, "Then how come you just spent the last hour staring at a stop sign?" I spent a Saturday afternoon at a high school soccer pitch in Cranbrook, B.C., taking shots at a former third-string goaltender for the Montreal Manic of the North American Soccer League, a French Canadian fellow named André Faggmann. He was, improbably, working for a few months on the railway gang to pass the summer before starting an MBA at U of T. He was hardly in need of my Frontier College services. I remember him punting the ball back to me just over the centre line, the ball rising in a gigantic arc, growing ever smaller then larger again as it descended from the high blue sky.

Beyond that, I tried to teach a large contingent of Sikh labourers to read in English. Then a band of nasty, thoroughly racist Albertan machine operators threatened to kick the shit out of me if I failed to organize a petition calling for the dismissal of one of the Sikh labourers because he had allegedly taken a dump in the Albertans' shower. As an act of self-preservation I did as I was told. And though I tarried sufficiently that the matter blew over, the Sikhs lost all interest in pursuing their studies with me.

But most of these happenings pale in my memory when set against the event that defined that summer. It occurred on a rainy early morning, before dawn. We were working on a stretch of rail outside Field, B.C., the foreman on our twenty-man crew of labes (short for labourers) an unhappy Italian drunk named Frank Longo. He had a long, gaunt, battle-weary face, the kind made famous in the wartime photography of Robert Capa. Rumour had it that he spent his evenings in his sleeping quarters on the train guzzling a combination of Scotch and NyQuil. He didn't take much of a shine to me, announcing early on that I was "the worst-a fuckin'-a labe" he'd seen in thirty years on the gangs. Oh dear.

On this particular morning Frank was—how to put it—a little on the surly side. Our crew had to change a long stretch of ties by hand. Usually, a couple of labes would be sent out ahead of the main crew to pull the spikes out of the ties and scatter the plates. That morning Frank put me—the slowest spike-puller on the gang—with Dervinder, a Sikh known as The Vinder, the fastest spike-puller on the gang. "And-a you better keep up or you gonna go home," said Frank. "Go home" was a euphemism for being fired.

So there I was, yanking spike after spike in the pouring rain, moving away from the main body of workers. Soon enough I was falling behind. And soon enough there was Frankie right in my face. "You better fuckin' hurry up or-a I'm gonna kicka you ass and you canna walk-a back to the train." (Twenty or so miles, as it happened.)

Then my luck changed. There appeared, as if conjured from the air, another labe. I remember him only as Frenchy. Frenchy scared the bejesus out of me. He was very short but incredibly muscular, far and away the strongest guy on the gang. He and I had struck up—I won't call it a friendship—let's say a mutual respect based on the fact that I found his Elmer Fudd impression startlingly funny. At any moment he might appear beside me and order me to be "vewy vewy quiet, I'm hunting wabbits."

At any rate, just after five a.m. with the rain streaming down our sky blue CPR helmets and in the glow of a single electric lantern that lit us from below, Frenchy turned to Frank and said, "Why don't you leave him the fuck alone?" And with that he didn't say another word but pitched in to help me catch up with The Vinder. I could see Frank's mouth working angrily, but there was nothing he could do since it was clear that, had he interfered, Frenchy, for reasons that probably had less than nothing to do with me, would have snapped him in two like a twig. Frenchy salvaged my dignity that day.

The other event that stays with me from that summer took place several thousand miles away, in the den of my parents' house in Rosedale. Mum was on the phone to a woman named Margaret Dalglish, who ran one of the major hospitals in London. Mother described her as "the Queen's nurse." I met her once years later, and she was the sort of Brit who reminds one that one has betters in this world. At any rate, mum was informing Margaret that her only son had gone to work for the Canadian Pacific Railway in the Rockies. As my mother tells it, there was a long pause and then, "Working on the rail . . . *way*. How . . . utterly . . . romantic." When my mother told me that story, full of love and admiration, I felt whole and ready for anything. It's weirdly ironic that I was only able fully to appreciate the idea of my noble purpose at two steps removed from my own experience. Only when mum felt comfortable with the idea, it having received the good aristocrat's seal of approval, and passed the word on to me did I feel an identification with my own actions. And they say the umbilical cord is cut at birth.

After an unmitigatedly disastrous turn at graduate studies in philosophy at McGill, the panic attacks worsened. Starting in the summer of 1984, I was working full-time for Frontier College in Toronto, where I remained for four years, through the first third of 1988. The attacks usually manifested themselves early in the morning. I would awaken suddenly with either pain in my chest or shortness of breath. My mind would immediately race from these ambiguous and half-imagined symptoms to a full-blown heart attack or aneurysm or whatever other physical disaster my imagination might conjure. It got to be so routine that a freshly minted girlfriend named Jean, a kindly, thoughtful law student, kept a batch of brown paper bags for me to breathe into so as to curtail my hyperventilating. The take on Jean, among my friends, was that she had to be a saint to put up with me.

I started seeing a psychiatrist in an effort to combat the effects of the attacks. I only ever seemed to discuss things that were bothering me at work—Frontier College office politics, etc. Sometimes I just made stuff up. Then I would tell the guy I was making stuff up and he wouldn't get upset. He'd just say, "Do you think that's helpful?" I always imagined this was a rhetorical question.

I thought I was making progress (I'd managed to get through several recent panic attacks without trooping down to Emergency), but I hadn't counted on the effect of returning to the scene of so much earlier upset: Florida. In the spring of 1986, I was invited by Jean's cousin Chris and a friend from Queen's to go on a tour of baseball spring training venues between Miami and West Palm Beach. I was reading a lot of baseball writing at the time (Thomas Boswell, Donald Hall, Daniel Okrent, Roger Angell and their ilk) and had a dreamy relationship to the game, one that included a passion for its tortured myths and analogies.

In fact, there wasn't anything terribly romantic about our tour, which was a week's worth of booze, rundown grapefruit league ballparks, and flirting with college girls on spring break. I spent one evening persuading a comely young thing from the University of North Carolina at

Chapel Hill that I was a consular officer with the British delegation in Miami, on the final night of my posting and in desperate need of ministrations only she could provide. I failed but congratulated myself for having sustained a competent Scottish brogue for the better part of four hours.

Every morning one or the other of our threesome threw up breakfast into the nearest potted palm. One night, midway through dinner in some crab shack or other, I wandered out onto the edge of a darkened waterway. Several large sailboats were moored along its concrete border. In a drunken fog, I stepped aboard one of the boats and began to rummage around in the cabin—pawing through family photos and letters. (I can't help but wonder whether I had a death wish, given the American penchant for shooting unwelcome visitors.) After I'd finished, I idled back to the crab shack, where I confessed my misadventure to my friends. They were too smashed to be shocked.

The next day we followed the pattern: breakfast, beach walk punctuated by potted palm pause, snooze. Then onto the golf course. There, on the eighteenth tee in Florida's reddish evening light, with a soft breeze smoothing my brow, I declared that I had never felt better in my life.

Later that night we decided to go to the dog races at Hollywood Park. These weren't just any dog races, mind, but the Super Bowl of American dog racing. As we clambered into the car and headed out onto the I95 (one of the busiest highways in America), I felt a wave of exhaustion wash over me. I checked my pulse. It was either too fast or too slow, I can't remember which. At any rate panic set in, followed hard on its heels by hyperventilation, which gave rise to tingling in my limbs, which in turn exacerbated the panic—*et voilà*, once again a lunatic was set upon the earth.

First I loosened the belt holding up my pants. Then I decided that if I was going to die, it would not be unremarked in the back of a car but flailing down a busy American highway in front of thousands upon thousands of rabid dog-racing aficionados. I popped open the back door and staggered several feet into the beams of, literally, thousands of headlights. My unbelted pants fell between my knees and I tripped. Then I passed out.

The consequence of my actions was sharp and swift. An ambulance and a cherry-top pulled up. The ambulance attendants asked if I was on cocaine while the cops searched the car and shook down my companions. (I learned later that in Florida at that time a BMW plus three white kids in Lacoste sports shirts equalled drug dealers.) From there it was off to Brouward County Hospital. It was ten-thirty on a Friday night, and the scene in the Emergency waiting room was like something from a *Frontline* documentary on inner-city violence. The patients were mostly black (and blue) and bleeding from every pore. A cop who, in manner and dress, reminded me of a prison guard in the film *Cool Hand Luke* looked across at us and drawled suggestively, "Boys, I think you-all've come to the wrong hospital."

In short order we were out the door and on our way to a private hospital in Pompano, somewhat nearer the privileged enclave where we were staying. The doctor who treated me, a puckish former Cuban refugee, judged that "maybe you need a vacation."

"I'm already on vacation."

"Maybe," he replied, "you need *another kind* of vacation."

A vacation, one supposes, from myself.

After we returned to Toronto, I called my pal from Queen's and asked him to keep my hysteria to himself.

"Uh-huh," he said, his voice betraying a certain skepticism. "How many people have you told already?"

"Hardly anyone," I lied sheepishly.

"The only reason you don't want me tell anyone is so you can keep the story for yourself."

And of course he was right. Delivered with the right mix of self-deprecation and absurdist humour, these yarns had comic potential. Usually the only one not laughing was Jean, who was contemplating a longer-term commitment to me. She always looked anxious and slightly mystified as to why I would find my own, oftentimes self-induced, propensity for ill health and hysteria so funny.

It was Super Sunday, January 25, 1987. Denver was to play the New York Giants in the NFL championship game. On the whole, my being was somewhat at odds with the prevailing superness. I had recently entered the world of full-time unemployment, having been relieved of my duties at Frontier College. (There's nothing so bracing for one's self-confidence as getting the axe from an ostensibly altruistic organization. You're actually not good enough to be, well, good.) I'd covered this ignominious fact by pretending to take another crack at graduate school, this time at York University. I was trying to qualify for an MA in environmental studies. Don't ask.

I had got quite drunk the night before, playing poker, and awoke feeling a bit sludgy. I decided to eat my way out of it. I consumed a variety of doughy pastries, overflowing with sweetened cherry and apple innards, and washed them down with too much coffee. Around lunch- time I felt a pressure radiating upwards from my solar plexus. I half sensed what was coming but, jittery with caffeine and sugar, decided to mistake acute pancreatitis for hunger. I made an enormous sandwich with pretty much everything I could find in the fridge and topped it off with a whipped-cream-like dollop of mayonnaise. As the pain increased, I tore into the sandwich with wolfish ardour. Then it was on me like a dog, sudden and intense.

I asked Jean to drive me to the hospital. On the way there I began to beat my fists inside the car. Jean asked me to calm down. I wondered: where does my pain end and my panic begin?

Inside the emergency room I was able to concentrate on my pain. Not that this made me any more stoic. I snapped at a nurse regarding the speed with which the results of my amylase test were being processed. There would be no relief till those tests were completed.

Then, just as suddenly as it had come over me, the pain dissipated. I remember thinking that I might even be able to carry on from the hospital to the Super Bowl party. No such luck. Dr. Allan Harrison was in charge of my care. He bluntly pointed out the unpleasant consequences of acute pancreatitis. Death, for one.

A couple of days later I received a visit in the hospital from a woman with whom I'd had sex several times over the previous couple of years. (This was in addition to a long-term relationship with Jean, who would become my wife.) We went down to the cafeteria for coffee, me marching along with my intravenous pole. I remember feeling distinctly uncomfortable, first because I was so obviously impaired by the pole and second because, despite the pole, I was so sexually aroused. We arrived back on the ward floor making very small talk. Suddenly she turned into a doorway off the hall, by the nursing station.

"You want to kiss me, don't you?"

I felt everything give way. "Uh-huh."

Somehow she directed me into an empty room, propped me on the side of a bed and unzipped my fly. Just as things were taking their natural upward and outward course, there was a commotion at the door. The back of a nurse's head poked around the corner. In that instant my friend moved up and off me, spat into a nearby closet and was on her way with a backward, singsongy "Byyyeee!"

Slipping past the nurse, who was backing into the room pulling a wheelchair, I scooted out hauling my IV pole. In retrospect what surprises me is how normal this all seemed; as if, under the circumstances, sexual congress was the expected response to hospitalization. Surrounded by every evidence of degeneration, my friend decided to stand up for generosity and vitalism. I'm probably somewhere between a stoic and a cynic, but for that moment the world appeared downright rosy.

Over the next couple of years I had a few relatively minor episodes of my pancreatic distress. Once, during a weekend at a resort near Collingwood, a gang of twenty or so friends spent the night with me at a local hospital. This led to a joke of sorts among that crowd:

Q. How does every story about Doug Bell end?
A. "Then he was rushed to the hospital."

PART 2

RUN OVER

GROWN UP

It is so very difficult for a sick man not to be a scoundrel.

— SAMUEL JOHNSON

"WHAT IS TO BE DONE?" asked Tolstoy, famously, about the poor. Axed by Frontier College, lacking even rudimentary self-confidence, hagridden by panic and with no real prospects, I decided, recklessly, to ask myself that same question.

Given my background and identity (or lack thereof), journalism seemed a nice compromise between the necessity of having some sort of professional realm into which one fit like a hand into a glove—all the questions answered before their posing, framing a sort of bespoke life for members of the entitled class—and actually seeking a way forward for myself. Of course journalism was a long way down the ladder from financier or lawyer or doctor or engineer, but it was something, a way to get from here to there—*there* being artistry, which in the minds of just about everyone I'd grown up with was highly suspect. Making art had to do with oneself, which meant one had to look within to find an answer as to the direction life could or should flow. Even as I write this, I feel a familiar knotting in my stomach. The notion of pursuing art in a self-conscious way still strikes me as pompous and annoying. Which leaves me feeling as though I'm pompous and annoying, which is no way to go through life.

At any rate, the transition from Frontier College and the comfortable sinecure of noblesse oblige liberalism to the point where I could even imagine life as a journalist had been slow. Jenny, a straightforward colleague at the college, noticed that I spent the better part of three years at my desk reading magazines. Serious, semi-serious, frivolous, I read it all: *The Nation*, *The New Republic*, the *Times Literary Supplement*, *The American Spectator*, *National Review*, *Spy*, *Private Eye*, *The New York Review of Books*, *Harper's*, *Tatler*, *Vanity Fair*, *The New Yorker*, *Washington Monthly*, *The National Review*, *Saturday Night*, *Business Week*, *Fortune*, *Canadian Business*. Magazines piled up around me like so much cordwood. I pretended that this had something to do with my job. "Why are you working here?" Jenny would ask incredulously. "You obviously want to be doing something else. You should get out and do it."

In my paranoid fashion I assumed she was trying to get rid of me. There's a distinctive push-pull that takes hold in the indecisive, insecure mind. Whatever your circumstances, they seem wholly imposed; at the same time, you are wholly to blame for your predicament. In therapeutic language this is known as dissociation. For me it's not so much a condition as a way of life. In the day-to-day course of things, as one is meant to be living in the moment, I have the sensation of waiting impatiently for something to happen over which I have little or no control. This sensation slowly builds to a point where, if only to relieve myself, I jerk higgledy-piggledy into motion, pursuing whatever it is that's just crossed my line of sight. But of course all that waiting leaves me with the sense that I've been wasting time, so there's the resulting impulse to rush, for fear that more time will pass waiting. Is that clear?

A concrete example might help. During the winter of 1987, when I was meant to be studying for a degree in environmental studies, I used to sit on the third floor of a house in Riverdale and while away the days pitching snowballs. I kept these snowballs on a blue and white china plate beside the couch. I would open the door to the deck a crack and try to pitch them through the opening. Sometimes, in a flurry of anxiety and fury, I'd pitch a high hard one and the snowball would explode over the door jamb, showering the carpet in snow. In the same moment my slow ticking anxiety would detonate and I would rush the length of the room to my desk, there to confront a pile of overdue books from the York University library. I would try to read, only to realize, mere seconds after starting, the abject futility of my efforts. Then it was back to the couch and the plate of snowballs.

Anyway, the result is more or less inevitable no matter the project, and soon enough the cycle starts up again. Sometimes I wonder whether my illnesses didn't give rise to a sort of macro version of my penchant for self-defeat. You wait to get sick because you know you will, inevitably, and in the meantime the rest of your life goes flying by, lost to you in the whirling distortions of your self-involvement.

Sometimes, though, the simple truth of an offhand observation like the one offered up by my friend Jenny takes hold and carries you through. And soon enough I was on the road away from do-gooding at Frontier College—towards what, I still wasn't sure.

In the late summer of my *annus snowbillus*, I pursued courses in publishing through the Banff Centre for the Fine Arts. Two of the courses (on computer and magazine publishing) took place in Banff, among the Rocky Mountains, and the third (in educational publishing) at Guelph University, in the midst of a staggering southern Ontario heat wave. The courses followed a workshop model, during which participants were split into groups of six and set more or less impossible publishing tasks, requiring more or less impossible standards of industriousness and sleeplessness. The faculty was made up entirely of industry pros who were looking to scout talent and scoop ideas, or so you were led to believe. For even the hardiest this was a pressurized environment. For me it was Dante's seventh circle of hell. One horribly sweaty night I went to bed very late with every conceivable conjecture passing through my mind, mostly of the if-I-screw-this-up-I'll-be-a-failure-for-life variety. After two hours of tossing and turning I gave up the ship and went into a full-blown panic. I had in my mind a half-remembered sleep disease that after seventy-two hours drives its victims into a coma and eventually kills them.

In my addled state I wandered the campus until sun-up, pausing to call Jean and then mum. The conversation with my mother was memorable mostly for her candour and sympathy. It was, after all, three in the morning. "Oh, you poor dear. Don't fret. Just get a book and read till you feel like falling asleep. I've had insomnia my whole life. I read and read and read. You've come by it honestly, though it's a terrible bore." I also remember conversing with two members of the cleaning staff, girlfriend-boyfriend, incredibly fit and healthy, ready-for-anything mountaineering types. In my scattered, anxious state I was a different species.

I went to the doctor as soon as the student health clinic opened. In addition to the usual questions regarding stress ("Stress . . . hmm, me? Yeah, I guess, I mean, sure, yeah. Stress, you say? Hmm . . . have you ever heard of this sleep disorder that kills you in seventy-two hours?") the doctor took my pulse, which was sufficiently elevated that she suggested I might want to take something that evening. She doled out a couple of white pills and sent me on my way.

The rest of the day is a bit of a blur except for a conversation with the program's director, a former sniper for an élite British commando unit who had often been forced to stay up forty-eight hours straight, waiting to make one shot. He didn't have much sympathy.

Later that evening, having exhausted warm milk, a diverting conversation and a good read, I turned to the pills. I downed them with a glass of water, then lay in my bed, panic's icy fingers beginning to play along my spine. All of a sudden Mum's words from the night before came to me. "I never sleep . . . you come by it honestly." And I felt warm and attached somehow to something, and a moment later I was asleep.

In the late spring of 1989, I married Jean. It was a happy day—lots of speeches, a big tent on the lawn hitched up to Jean's parents' place in Ottawa; plenty of champagne, dancing, falling over, men (who otherwise wouldn't) hugging each other; all capped by a judge across the street calling the cops to shut things down. Perfect.

I had asked for Jean's hand the previous summer under an oak tree alongside the Washington Monument in the city of her birth. I had started into a job that I thought would lead me towards writing as a life. I was a sub-editor at a business magazine—to my mind the most stressful, challenging job available to a Western male. Jean seemed born to the task of supporting me in the tortured and tortuous effort to establish myself. She was kind, her expression gentle and her colouring the most beautiful I'd ever seen. The skin around her eyes was particularly arresting, flecked as it was with light purples and blues. Her pale blue eyes were like twin suns.

Her mother was Flemish, from Ostend. Her maternal grandfather had known and patronized the Flemish painter James Ensor, whose deeply subversive work—rooted in the mad satires of Bosch and Daumier—I had admired even before meeting Jean. (Her father endeared himself to me by commenting on Ensor's work, "God, he's a cynical bastard.") Her great-grandfather had been a leading figure in the Belgian socialist party. For whatever reason, Belgian socialism struck me as terribly exotic. Jean represented what a friend of mine, a discerning Winnipeg Jew, recently described as "all the qualities of highly civilized society."

Beyond that, Jean provided a buffer to my mother's smothering concern. First, she was terribly bright and professionally accomplished, and second, she was very tall. In my barely adolescent brain I imagined that these factors might intimidate my mother enough that she'd cut me a little slack.

Furthermore, I had a vague sense that, yes, my "life's work" had to do with words, but because of my natural disinclination to competent endeavour and good health I needed a steady source of income.

All this was set against my relentless need to curry mother's favour, which I would seek whether I had any currency to bargain with or not. In lean times I would simply cut a pattern from whole cloth: TV shows I'd been invited to appear on, short lists made, jobs offered and rejected. Artful exaggeration was the hallmark of our shared conversational strategies. There is of course a healthy dose of self-delusion that accompanies the will to fib for effect. Whenever mother would produce a whopper, I would put both hands together and wave them in a swimming motion. This was a short form for what I had dubbed my mother's tunas (as in "look at the size of the tuna that just swam by"). In response mum would invariably feign shocked indignation.

I too was subject to public upbraiding for my fish tales. Even at university I noticed that, as I declaimed on some subject or other, certain of my friends would start stabbing their right index fingers into the palms of their left hands. I eventually asked one of them, "What the fuck are you doing?"

"I'm calculating the Doug Bell expansion factor."

I measured myself against everyone whose work I respected or thought I ought to respect. Their destinies seemed so clear to me: onward and upward to greatness, achievement and fame. Why couldn't I see my future as clearly and forcefully? That's where Jean came in. She would save me from my failures, from my flawed sense of self. She'd be me, only better. All I had to do was show up and marry her—not exactly how they draw it up in the matrimonial playbook.

In the spring of 1990, I found myself fighting nagging stomach pains at work. I put this down to panic arising from the stress of editing a magazine devoted to business without a clue how to balance my own chequebook.

Among the legion of panic attacks that dotted my psychic landscape, perhaps my favourite of all time occurred in the midst of a squash match in early 1990. I had not properly hydrated, and in the heat of competition I began to feel light-headed and weak. At the conclusion of the match I thought I might faint. Panic set in, and the combination of these various conditions (some real, some imagined) combined to put me into a tailspin.

My complaints brought the club manager and eventually a doctor, who'd been upstairs having dinner. I lay against the lockers in the men's changing room, swathed in wet towels. The doctor took my wrist authoritatively in his hand to check my pulse. My heart continued to whack away at 150 beats per minute. I asked what he thought might be the matter. He looked at me and in a hearty voice meant to reassure said, "No idea really, I'm a gynecologist. Probably best that we call in an ambulance and you go to the hospital just to be on the safe side." I actually started to laugh.

While I was rolled out to the awaiting ambulance, I saw the mother of a friend who I knew was on the club's board. For some reason I imagined that making a scene like this was in contravention of club rules. As if to mitigate the damage, I piped up in a hail-fellow-well-met brogue, "Uh, oh hi, Mrs. Knowles, not to worry just a spot of bother no need to fret or feel that you need to *tell* anyone about this." I babbled all the way out the door while Mary Knowles trailed behind, murmuring her condolences.

"Right then," I said cheerily as the attendants closed the ambulance doors. "Byeee!"

At the magazine it seemed that everyone had either quit or just plain buggered off. Everyone, that is, save me. The editor-in-chief had been the subject of an internal coup d'état launched by the publisher. This came on top of a situation involving a staff editor who assigned a column he had no power to commission, let alone run, to a writer for whom he had sexual ambitions. After several months of inventing excuses for the column's non-appearance ("We had to take it out just as we were going to press. There was a reference in there to a plane crash and the column turned out to be running opposite an ad for one of the airlines. Well, we couldn't have that . . .") he was accosted by the writer in his office. I happened to be there at the time and remember slouching further and further into the editor's couch while he ran through his roster of excuses, my stomach twisted up like a wet towel ready to be snapped.

As it turned out, I was able to untangle myself from this disaster by finding a new job as an editor for a supplement to *The Globe and Mail*, and I even managed to wangle a week off between jobs. For the first time in what I laughingly referred to as my career in journalism, my parents seemed at least to have heard of a publication that was willing to hire me, though my mother offered her standard response to my peripatetic career course: "Well, it's all good experience." Every time she said this I wanted to grab her by the lapels: "For Christ's sake, experience for what ? This is it. This is what I do. This isn't experience, this is it, this is what I want to do. Why do you keep saying that?" I think now that she believed, no matter what stock you put in work or love or redemption, life in the end will let you down. Granted—but what I needed was the tried and true: tell the kid he's God's gift to the orb and let the poor beggar find out the truth for himself.

I arrived home after my last day at the old job, having more or less edited an entire issue by myself. Rather than luxuriate in the prospect of a week off, I ricocheted around the house in a blind rage, smashing several lamps and a couple of chairs. Though too terrified to see my situation for what it was (I imagined my anger had something to do with overwork), somewhere beneath the neat rationalizations and outright lies I knew I was staring into the abyss. I'd been drinking and popping 222s to cover the pain that was blanketing my waking life, and the only thing I wasn't dulling was the truth.

Two days later I took off to Vancouver. The plan was for Jean to follow me, and then we would fly to Seattle and take a road trip down the Pacific coast all the way to San Francisco.

That first day in Vancouver held such promise. I collected several newspapers in the morning, then went to breakfast and down to Kitsilano beach to lie with my back propped on a driftwood log while I read of Saddam Hussein's adventures in Kuwait. Later I walked west through the wooded UBC campus and over to the anthropology museum, where I wandered among the tribal totems of Canada's Pacific northwest.

After that I sauntered to the edge of the museum's grounds to stare out at the ocean, and then took the steep stairway to a beach below, stumbling the last few steps onto the sand. I know I must have heard about Wreck Beach, but there's something too delicious about wandering aimlessly and uninformed to let prior knowledge dilute the joy of discovery. I was wearing a buttoned-down shirt, khakis and a pair of brown suede brogues. I removed my shoes and socks and rolled up my pants. For some reason I was reminded of a *Doonesbury* cartoon depicting Richard Nixon, shortly after his resignation, walking on the beach at San Clemente with a metal detector.

Once again I propped myself against a log and started reading. A shadow fell over me. I lifted my right hand to my brow in a sort of naval salute. This cut the glare from the early afternoon sun bouncing off the Pacific chop. Standing before me, shining oily brown and utterly naked, was a man sporting a wispy growth of beard and a quizzical look. "Beer?" he said.

I was confused.

I looked directly at his penis while I stumbled over a response. "Uh...yeah...sure...okay." I fumbled around in my pants pocket for my...money. I pulled out sheaves of loose papers, Kleenex, a golf tee and various rumpled two-dollar bills. The man squinted disapprovingly at this mess and reached into my mitt to remove the right amount. Behind him two men *sans culottes* sauntered past lazzarone-like, their sunglass eyes taking in the scene. The man in front of me reached behind him into one of those metallic-coloured pliable coolers and produced a beer. He handed it to me and walked quickly away down the beach after the two who had just passed by. His heels dug into the sand, producing little sprays of grit with each step.

I was staying on my friend Mike's couch, and when I got home I told him the story as though I'd seen a steady stream of flying midgets taking off in formation from the Vancouver airport. Mike gave a so-what shrug and I was left with an uncomfortable feeling. It's how I feel whenever my "funny" stories fall flat, somewhere between "Fuck you" and "I'm terribly sorry."

The next morning I was awakened by a dull but persistent pain in my gut. I met Jean at the airport to catch our connecting flight to Seattle, complaining of the steady pain. She sensibly suggested that we seek medical attention in Vancouver before heading off into the American health care wilderness. However, I was determined not to succumb to my fear.

The flight down to Seattle was agonizing. I felt at once flushed and clammy. By the time we arrived, I was into the first of a series of short bursts of relief that persuaded me the worst was over. In Seattle, Jean rented a large luxury car, the kind pimps drove in 1970s American cop shows. It had a gauge that allowed constant monitoring and adjustment of the temperature inside the car, a mechanism that would figure prominently over the next few days.

We drove downtown, parked, and wandered among Seattle's caffeine-addled citizenry. Later we walked out to the hideously concrete domed stadium to take in a Mariners game. The pain that had dogged me on the plane came back. In my usual fashion I decided to fight fire with gasoline. At the concession stand I bought some sort of pig-fat monstrosity. Jean gasped at the sight of it. I downed it. Later we wandered around Pioneer Square, part of a snaking caravan moving back from the ballpark, the sounds of Seattle's music scene drifting out of the doorways of clubs packed tight. I felt fine again.

Just before dawn my discomfort pushed me out of oblivion. I headed for the common room at our bed and breakfast and sat watching the light move across Puget Sound. I knew I was in trouble. The pain ebbed slightly as we headed out onto Highway 1. As we drove, I pushed the temperature around in concert with my thermal fluctuations. "Too hot . . .too cold . . . too hot," I'd mumble, flipping up to eighty-five and back to sixty as we made our way down the coast. Finally, Jean reached over and touched my forehead with the back of her hand. "Doug," she said in the infinitely patient tone she's always used with me, "you've got a fever." We stopped in Aberdeen, Washington, to pick up a thermometer so I could at least monitor the temperature that mattered.

As we headed for the Grays Harbor Community Hospital, it became clear to us that Aberdeen must have been the model for Twin Peaks, David Lynch's fictional logging town. In Emergency there was a longish wait as a series of logging calamities were dealt with—severed digits and the like. The doctor who eventually listened to my history took a blood test to determine whether my amylase was elevated. It wasn't. By the time the results came back from the lab, my fever had dropped. Another reprieve, a bit like a stay of execution. I took it to mean more than it did, more than it could.

We carried on down the coast. I was sore but happy. I studied the map and imagined what it might be like to drive into Mendocino, north of San Francisco. There was a song by Kate and Anna McGarrigle *(Talk to me of Mendocino/ closing my eyes I hear the sea...)*. I imagined a place evocative enough to give rise to a lyric as beautiful as that, and hummed the song to myself as we drove along in the dimming light of the Oregon coast. We decided to stop in a place called Newport, settled into a seaside motel and watched, of all things, a rerun of *Twin Peaks*. Jean kept asking how I was doing. I continued to feel clammy, but there was little or no pain. The stay seemed to be holding.

The next day we awoke and went looking for one of those authentic American spots, the sort of eatery described by Jack Kerouac in *On the Road*: "There were seafood places where the buns were hot, and the baskets good enough to eat too; where the menus themselves were soft with foody esculence as though dipped in hot broths and roasted dry and good enough to eat too." We picked a place that sat on the end of a pier, not unlike the spots we might have seen on Fisherman's Wharf if we had made it to Fisherman's Wharf.

As we began to eat, I felt the now familiar discomfort begin to build. Jean noted my desperate ferocity and told me to ease off on the food. That only drove me to shove the greasy mash of eggs, toast, bacon and jam deep down my gullet. Years later I got swarmed by gypsy kids on the Arbat in Moscow, their little hands moving inside my every pocket, every opening. It reminded me of the onset of pancreatitis. It's not so much that the pain is inside you as you're inside the pain, just like the little gypsy hands aren't so much inside your pockets as you are inside the swarm.

Jean and I got into the car and went back to the motel. Her inquiries became more urgent and my rebuffs curter. I was deluded enough to think that simply lying down would help. I remember the morning light piercing my eyes as I walked towards the room, and having to turn back to the car and ask Jean to head for the hospital. Then something let go in me and I was banging around the car like an angry bee inside a jar. Jean was driving too slowly. She was driving too fast. My fists smashed against the dashboard and on the ceiling. But for all that, the world was retreating.

We got to Emergency and I was admitted immediately. I remember asking everyone I came in contact with how soon I might get a shot for the pain. Understandably, doctors want to see evidence of some malfunction in the body to justify their diagnosis and subsequent action; writhing isn't enough. The pain, I realize now, wasn't fierce enough yet to knock out that part of my rational mind that could still follow the process.

The blood tests came back and, though they still didn't indicate the source of the pain, my behaviour must have finally done the trick. I was referred to an internist and given a shot of Demerol. I don't remember the amount, but it didn't have the usual effect. The pain was still there like an insistent sound; though growing fainter, it promised havoc on its return.

Near midday I was taken up onto a ward, where I fell into an all-black sleep. When I awoke, it was to another stay of execution, but I felt weaker, as if I had only the governor's clemency left to rely on, all other appeals having been exhausted. The internist, Dr. Gary Thueson, turned up. He was weedy and uncertain. I ascertained that he'd attended medical school at Brigham Young University, a Mormon college in Utah with an excellent football program. (When I mentioned this, he didn't seem to know what I was talking about.) Nothing else he said imbued me with confidence. He scheduled a test in which some radioactive fluid would pass into my digestive system. He would follow it on a screen. This would tell him something.

The next afternoon a nurse came in to check my temperature, and she looked . . . odd. She was almost freakishly bony, and the bones seemed to stick out of her at all sorts of weird angles. She held her upper arms out rigidly at forty-five degrees from her torso. Her forearms dangled loosely, her palms facing away like the Scarecrow's in *The Wizard of Oz*.

"This is okay," I thought, trying for hysterical optimism. "I'm sure she's competent."

She addressed me in a terrifyingly slushy staccato. "I'm shupposed to. . .I've got tchew . . . I'm going to take your tchemperatchure."

"That's okay," my courageous inner voice announced. "Whatever her appearance, she clearly knows what she's doing. Hiring the physically impaired for this kind of work is the right thing to do."

She was beside the bed now, struggling with something. It turned out to be a digital-readout thermometer, the kind they stick in your ear. She scrunched over, trying to get the sterile cap onto the tip of the thermometer. Suddenly there was an eruption of physical force and my bed was showered in little sterile caps.

"Got it," she announced, triumphant, as the caps settled on the bed around me. "Now, how does this work?" she pondered as she began to stick the thermometer at various parts of my earlobe, missing the canal that might tell both of us what we needed to know.

I began to babble nervously. "Look, maybe you should get somebody else in here—your . . . your . . . boss, supervisor, the head nurse or somebody."

She maintained a sort of rictus grin. "It's okay. We'll just do it the old way."

She jammed a mercury thermometer under my tongue and went about her business. Unable to speak, I glanced around the room wild-eyed, looking for someone who might save me.

Later in the afternoon I started to hurt, and this time I was afraid even before the pain really took hold. It occurs to me that I received two doses of painkiller, one orally and the other injected, the one on top of the other. The moment this cocktail began to take effect, I sensed something was off.

I was flashing hot and cold. Jean was in the room at the time and it was clear that her resources were depleting under the onslaught of my upset. It took the better part of two hours for me to calm down.

Later that day I was taken down for the radioactive diagnostic. It was a weekend and the Pacific Communities Hospital of Newport, Oregon, was a morgue. The procedure seemed to take forever. I felt ill and alone and a long way from home. At some point whatever it was they were tracing through my system stopped, indicating a blockage of some kind. As it was the weekend, I would have to wait till the next morning to discover my fate.

That night I saw a very large Samoan fellow (a navy man, as it turned out) being wheeled out to a helicopter that had landed on the hospital helipad. He had contracted a rare tropical disease and they were taking him to a specialized military hospital where his condition could be treated more effectively. I longed to go with him.

Thueson turned up the next day and announced that the tests indicated there was something wrong with my gallbladder. He thought I had gallstones and was referring me to a surgeon to discuss a course of action. This struck me as equivalent to a tree surgeon suggesting that a pile of firewood was suffering from Dutch elm disease and bringing in a specialist to try and save the tree. Through the rest of that day Jean and I discussed our options. With hindsight the first option should have been to clear out of Dodge.

As it turned out, Dr. Richard K. Beemer looked like the answer to our prayers. He was square-jawed with close-cropped steel grey hair. He had an easy, confident manner. He assured me that for twenty years he'd been practising exactly the sort of surgery I would require. So far, so good.

"We'll wait to see how you're doing in the morning. If things aren't going well, we'll pop out your gallbladder. I've done a lot of these things. I'm even planning to keep my date with the boys over at the volunteer fire department. We'll have a few beers, tell a few stories. And I'll still be in shape to drop over in the morning and take out your gallbladder, if need be."

As Dr. Beemer blithely continued to fill us in on the finer points of his schedule, I found my eyes shifting beseechingly to Jean's.

"Um, could I maybe just have a quick word with my wife . . . in private?"

What followed was a panicky series of conversations and telephone calls involving my parents and Dr. Harrison in Toronto. I remember the Oregon doctor saying to Harrison over the phone, "I've been doing this for twenty-five years. I'm confident of my diagnosis." Beemer then handed the phone over to me. Harrison's middle-Ontario drawl indicated nothing save the incontrovertible fact of his preference. "I think it would be best if you flew back to Toronto as soon as possible."

Beemer left after that phone call, with the promise he'd be back first thing in the morning and "we'll deal with it then." Jean stayed for a while. She'd been in touch with my parents, who were sending along first-class air tickets for a flight the next morning. For once I in no way begrudged my parents' help.

Soon enough, Jean was headed back to her motel for the night. Stranded on my bed after she left I felt an immense helplessness, as though I were bobbing lost in calm waters just as the wind began to rise and the ocean to sway.

"There are no atheists in foxholes. There are no atheists in foxholes. There are no atheists in foxholes." I kept repeating this like a mantra throughout the night. It seemed my inner voice was asking God to spare my life in return for improved future performance. It was all I could do to keep the darkness at bay. Illness as an adolescent is about pain; illness as an adult is about regret.

I listened to every click and whirr emanating from the hospital through those hours, and every click and whirr mocked me. In a day, a week, a year, those sounds would signal a patient's health restored, and in turn that patient restored to lover, spouse and children. Would I be so restored? I didn't know, and that scared the living shit out of me. So I whiled away the dark hours bargaining with the Almighty.

In the morning I awoke like a man who hadn't slept. A greasy wash of flop sweat sloshed between the furrows of my forehead. I sensed my body failing me like a debtor ducking a creditor's call. A while later, in popped the aptly named Dr. Beemer. "You look fine," he said, his white teeth flashing, full of confidence, "right as rain."

Moments earlier I'd stepped out of the bathroom, having examined my pallor under the hideous flourescent light so favoured of prisons and hospitals. "Gawd, you're practically green," I'd thought. Hard on the heels of that observation came the realization that the reason I *looked* green was that I was in fact *turning* green. I'd seen it fifteen years earlier at Sick Kids, when a nurse held a mirror to my face in the intensive care unit: the whites of my eyes had turned yellow. Though less vivid, the same process was underway now. This thought, or something awfully close to it, occurred to me as Dr. Beemer finished his peppy summation.

"Look," I said, pulling the flesh away from one eye.

"Nope," the doctor intoned in a happy timbre, "I don't see it." At which point he gave me a bunch of painkillers with vague instructions as to their use and withdrew with a hearty wave. But not before laying the following all-American odds: "You're fine to fly," he said. "It's a million to one that anything's gonna go wrong on that flight."

As we passed through the lush agricultural lands between Newport and Portland on the way to the airport, the industrial sprinklers released a torrent of artificial rain into the muggy air. I remember leaning out of the car's open door at a crossroads with four perfectly square fields stretching away from each corner. I threw up, though in my weakened condition the bilge more or less fell out of me like so many coins from an inverted pocket. By the time we got to the airport, Jean was nervous and I was cranky yet strangely resigned. Jean suggested that maybe we ought to find a teaching hospital in Portland, though we didn't know if one existed. But we were getting down to the wire for our flight, and what with the panicky arrangements we were unsure of our fate should we miss it. We ploughed on.

In the lounge by the gate I began to experience the pain circling inside my trunk. It felt huge. But I was way out beyond the north boundary of wishful thinking and into the realm of lottery players listening to the radio for the winning number. By the time the plane started to taxi for takeoff, all I had left of my hope was a torn-up ticket. I realized that for the next three hours at least (the length of time it takes to fly from Portland to Chicago, where we were meant to change planes for Toronto) I was going to feel as though I were being eaten alive from the inside out.

Now, there are certain things I can be grateful for even as I write an account of the worst hours of my life to date (yes, including the accident). First, accompanying us on the plane that day was Dr. James McCann of Wabash, Indiana, who restored my faith in the medical profession. Second, my wife was a calming, heroic presence who had the courtesy and good breeding not to fall apart till after the situation had resolved itself. Third, I lived.

Twenty minutes after takeoff I was on the phone from the plane to Beemer's office in Newport. I was in such a state that I'd have called him just to remind him of those million-to-one odds he'd offered up with such confidence ("What's the payoff on those odds, doc? Cash? Chips maybe? Or how about three hours of screaming misery?"). But in fact, I had some serious questions concerning the painkillers he'd handed out. He'd given us Tylenol Three and Percodan, and since the Tylenol was like pitching underhand to Sammy Sosa, we were wondering when I should move up the sliding analgesic scale to Percodan. Of course, in the event, I forced Jean to give me a Percodan shortly after the Tylenol proved ineffective. So the call was actually more an effort to discover how much damage I might already have done.

Jean began on the phone with an effort to remain calm. Her tone was reasonable: *Houston, we have a problem.* "Doug's in an awful lot of discomfort and we were just wondering . . ."

In that moment the pain took hold of me like a shark with one of those sides of beef they drop underwater to drive the poor creature to frenzy. I grabbed the phone. "Look, I just took a Percodan right on top of Tylenol. Is that a problem?"

The voice on the other end of the phone had an ever so slightly indignant I-simply-don't-have-time-for-this tone. "Look, ah, I *suppose* you *could* stop breathing."

The shark continued to sink his teeth in, wrenching me this way and that. Somewhere inside the black pit where my darker demons stir, a light went on. I turned to Jean and said, "Way to go, you just killed me." Charming, no?

Even so, Jean did her best to keep me calm. For the next forty minutes or so I vomited all over the first-class cabin. Anything that might have killed me ended up on the carpet or on the shoes of a fellow passenger.

For a time I felt the pain was my own, no need to share it. I remember moaning gently along with the engine's throbbing beat. Then, suddenly, there he was, my angel from Wabash, Indiana, Dr. James McCann. He had gentle hands and a kind manner, matter-of-fact when he needed to be, gentle the rest of the time, just like any good doctor. And he got it right first time. "You're having an attack of acute pancreatitis. Your abdomen's still soft, so you're not in any immediate danger. I know the pain must be horrible. Just hang on. I'm calling ahead to Chicago. They'll pick you right up off the runway. Don't worry, just hang in there."

Throughout the trip I had been conscious of the stiff faces of my fellow passengers. Like all good WASPs faced with a scene—a couple fighting at the next table, Jews weeping at the thought of the Holocaust, or a man vomiting harum-scarum throughout the first-class cabin all the way from Portland to Chicago—best to ignore it, dear. And for this I am grateful. What sort of horror might have ensued had someone actually taken exception to my booting like a college drunk for the better part of two hours?

As the plane taxied along the runway at O'Hare airport, I saw the flashing lights of an ambulance and an accompanying cop car sliding out to meet us. I imagined the first-class passengers standing at a respectful distance whispering words of comfort to my wife, maybe even a smattering of admiring applause as I was wheeled off. In the event, the impatient mob of hard-faced Yankees rushed the door. The stewardesses pushed back, asking them please to wait for the paramedics to get the young man off the plane. I heard my sensible, mild and cerebral wife tell some Midwestern matriarch to "Back up, will ya!? Back up." She wouldn't.

As I stood stooped under the overhead baggage bin, I felt the ocean surge of bodies pushing forward and then, caught by the undertow, swaying back. Out of some primordial flare for the dramatic I decided my best bet was to crawl between the writhing, entwined figures surrounding me. As I moved forward on all fours through the stockinged underbrush, I looked up and caught the eye of a paramedic in a blue uniform. "Is it you?" he asked. The shark wagged his head insistently. "Yeah," I groaned, "it's me."

Strapped onto the stretcher, slipping down the side-exit stairs from the gangway, I saw first the pink streaks of cloud in the sky over the dead flat Illinois horizon, then the ridged pattern on the roof of the ambulance, and finally the long fluorescent bulbs in the hospital hallway slipping by like a dotted line on the highway. I felt as though I were moving from one level of illness to another, pulling the pain around me like a cloak. Only one thought now: kill the pain . . . kill the pain . . . kill the pain.

After Newport, the Emergency nurses were a huge improvement, big-city quick and efficient. Direct looks, direct answers. Still, I took little comfort in this.

A doctor turned up, as square-jawed as Dr. Beemer but with earnest, intelligent eyes.

"Look, I know it's pancreatitis," I told him. "The doctor on the plane, McCann, he wrote it down. I need morphine, Demerol, something."

The doctor looked at me evenly. "We need to take your blood and get the results from the lab before we make any decisions."

This wasn't the answer I wanted to hear. My needs were primitive and I responded accordingly. "Aw, for Christ's sake, we both know what those fucking tests are going to show. Either the amylase isn't going to show up or it is. Either way I'm still fucked, so give me the fucking shot."

The doctor's eye narrowed. "We'll proceed as I've instructed."

"Fuck you," I spat.

The doctor held my eyes for a moment, anger playing at the corners of his mouth, and then marched out behind the curtain without a further word. (For the most part doctors don't understand that patients get angry when they feel pain. I suspect they believe that anger is an irrational response to whatever efforts they're making to alleviate the pain. But that's not the point; the pain itself is the issue.) Several moments later the doctor was back, having softened his tone. I babbled an apology out of the desperate need to feel that things were continuing to move forward.

Later, an older nurse with a gentle expression turned up by my bed. I was barely able to hold my eyes open. She looked at my chart and her expression brightened. "I see here you've been assigned to Dr. Meccia. He's good. I think he owns the Emergency. He's highly motivated to keep you alive."

"Sweet shit," I responded, it being the only thing I could think of to say.

The nurse looked confused for a moment, then patted my hand. "You rest now, honey."

I finally got my shot and the pain receded like a very loud noise that has moved a little out of range. The treatment for acute pancreatitis is fairly simple. Using a vacuum pump, draw out all of the digestive juices from the belly through a tube inserted into the stomach through the nose. These juices run out into a large bell-shaped jar beside the bed. The hope is that by shutting down all digestive activity in the abdomen, the pancreas will be tricked into shutting itself down. This is a bit like the Soviet solution to the Chernobyl crisis: encase the whole flaming mess in a concrete sarcophagus and hope the problem goes away. There is, after all, nothing else to do.

On that first night Jean sat by the bed on the ward and watched my fitful sleep. Late in the evening she decided to take a nap in her room. At four in the morning she woke and, full of restless energy, decided to come see me. Jean was staying in a wing of the hospital reserved for transients caught up in the health disasters of friends and relatives. She was in her nightie, housecoat and slippers. As she moved to the elevator, she fidgeted with her key. Because she was tired and agitated, her fingers failed her and the key was launched from her hand. Turning through space, it landed between the edge of the floor and the elevator door, and slipped down the shaft. Jean could hear the diminishing sound of the key as it deflected on its way down. "PLINK, ping, ding, d'ding, ding..." Just then a nun came round the corner and, seeing the look on Jean's face, rushed to her side. It was as if her life were falling away from her down a bottomless well.

My most vivid memory from that first night falls somewhere between perception and hallucination. When sleep comes under the influence of painkillers, it does so in fits and starts. Despite the muffling effect of the Demerol, the brain, even in repose, needs to fit the pain into some context so as to make sense of it. I suspect it's a bit like the ringing alarm clock that enters your dream first thing in the morning. The dream's storyline will alter suddenly to accommodate the insistent sound. Doped up on Demerol, the pain is the equivalent of the alarm, only you don't ever quite wake up.

That night I dreamed I was a head of state or someone with grave responsibilities. The pain was a sort of inequity I was required to rectify, but there were many complications. Every time I thought I was near a solution, some complication would arise and I'd be right back where I started. I remember at one stage I felt I had to sign some sort of document, a contract or treaty of sorts. I was aware of moving my hand as though signing my name. Then, a moment later, someone was standing in the doorway, shouting, and I was set upon by a gaggle of nurses. What I imagined as signing my name the nurses saw as the hallucinatory behaviour of a deranged patient waving around the business end of a nasogastric tube and depositing its contents on the clean white sheets of his bed.

The next morning I met a Dr. Bransfield. He had a *brad Chicahgo ahccent*, his vowels opening up like barn doors. His hair was buzz-cut marine. He listened to my abdomen with a stethoscope and grimaced. He didn't pull any punches. "Let's hope your bowels start working or else you're in trouble." Before I had time to ask what this might mean, he was gone.

I was left in the care of a busty, equally matter-of-fact nurse with a fabulously Polish name I couldn't begin to pronounce, let alone remember. She changed the linens around my limp form, hoisting me up and down off the bed like a rag doll. She was the one who explained the implications of having no activity in the bowels. It wasn't good.

As that day wore on, I became sufficiently aware of things to notice that next to me in the room was a man in his middle fifties who was having an operation for stomach cancer. He shuffled around in slippers, pyjamas and a ratty housecoat, a defeated expression on his chinless face. The sad pouches under his eyes fell away and hung in mid-air like climbers suspended from the face of a cliff. One of his kids turned up, slouching around in a leather jacket, bumming a smoke and looking bored, a dead ringer for Joey Ramone.

That afternoon I felt the slight pressure of pooling gas in my lower abdomen and, sure enough—yes!—a fart. I practically shouted with glee as the faintly sulphurous odour reached my nostrils. Imminent death was averted.

Later, a Cubs game appeared on local television. I carried on a lively (or as lively as might be expected from two men lying flat on their backs with no prospect of getting up anytime soon) conversation with my roommate regarding the Cubs' chances. Things seemed reassuringly normal. Jean arrived and, though she has no interest in baseball, sat by the bed kneading my hand as I focused on balls, strikes, hits and outs—the diverting details of America's pastime.

Then the pain came back to remind me who was slave, who master. My body was like a pointless misanthropic teenager doing damage for no reason beyond the sheer thrill of destruction. My pancreas was a vandal smashing the furniture, spray-painting obscenities on the curtains and taking a shit in the bathtub. "And what," my body seemed to scream, "are you gonna do about it?"

I got another shot and the baseball game melted away from me, the action on the screen just a series of images flickering in a distant corner of the room. Far away in the other corner, I twisted from side to side, looking deeper and deeper inside my pain and finding no sense and no relief.

The next morning I awoke with little or no discomfort, and for a brief time the absence of pain was a tonic verging on the erotic. It was wonderful just to feel the physical outline of myself, stretching the muscles in my legs, arching my back for the heck of it. Experiencing my corporeal self without having to make sense of it. Feeling nothing for its own sake.

Shortly thereafter, my mother blew in from Toronto. The worst had passed, but in her usual fashion Mum thought it important that I be treated as though a full-blown crisis were still in progress; only in this way could the full importance of her son be properly recognized. Mum had made a request through the Ontario government that I be transported by air ambulance from Chicago to Toronto, the only proviso being that the surgeon in charge of my care sign off. This turned out to be Dr. Meccia, the fellow who owned Emergency. After a morning in which I was treated to a full-body CAT scan, which turned up nothing but did give me a fabulous photo of my innards (Doug's Summer Vacation), Dr. Meccia scheduled a "conference" to discuss my options. Despite my every encouragement for her to get out and see Chicago ("The Wrigley building is supposed to be great, mum, you really should see it. And what about the Art Institute while you're at it?"), my mother insisted on sticking around. "I won't utter," she promised, which for her was the equivalent of the old Hollywood saw that "if they say it's not about money, believe me, it's about money."

Meccia turned up bedside and started explaining the ins and outs of pancreatitis to me. Along with him was some junior distaff version of the boss. Meccia wore a starched white lab coat with his signature stitched over the breast pocket. He and his assistant both sported chunky, thick-rimmed glasses that gave them goggle eyes. As he spoke, he would squint in a slightly annoyed fashion every now and then, as if to ask, "Aren't you getting this? I'm not sure you're getting this." His assistant mimicked the look without the voice-over.

Meccia drew a bunch of diagrams that I was to take back with me to the doctors in Toronto. Maybe he imagined that Canadian doctors needed the diagrams to understand the diagnosis adequately (the same diagnosis that Dr. James McCann had come up with without even a stethoscope). Irrationally, I decided to try to enlist Meccia in my condemnation of the Oregon doctors. ("Hey, they were incompetent, right? I mean, they were really incompetent, right?") Meccia was evasive. The assistant stared hard at me with eyes that, magnified by her lenses, looked to be the size of manhole covers.

At this point mum decided it was time to turn a sticky situation into a quagmire. She launched in on the air ambulance, her voice taking on an imperious tone that shifted towards imperious anger the more steadfast Dr. Meccia became in his refusal to countenance the idea. "This is absolutely unacceptable. This child has been grievously ill. What if he's ill again on the flight?" The second I heard that word *child* (I was thirty years old), I saw red. Meccia looked blankly at my mother. Then he said something about taking her views under advisement and left.

In a voice I remember as being low and weirdly intense even to my own ears, I told Jean that if she didn't get my mother out of my hair, I would do something drastic. Luckily, Jean was able to distract mum long enough to get her downtown.

We flew back to Toronto on a regularly scheduled commercial flight. I remember stretching out on the seats in the lounge while waiting to board, thumbing through the *Chicago Tribune*. The warm, late August sun beamed through O'Hare's glass and painted steel. I was weak but alive, and just then that seemed good enough for me.

At Sunnybrook my situation was more or less ideal. I was in a private room in a hospital where those most responsible for my care knew I was the direct descendant of the hospital's most prominent and successful chairman, and an heir of the family that had owned the land on which the hospital was situated. Convalescing in these circumstances had a Janus-faced quality, an entitlement issue on a rather grand scale. On the one hand I felt as though I had a right to take whatever time I needed to re-establish my sense of well-being. On the other hand, that "right" born of privilege was wholly fictitious. My body would react how it bloody well pleased, and no amount of belief in my special status as a focus of concern for the doctors and nurses would change that. As a result, I felt guilty for taking perhaps more time recovering than I would have had I been an ordinary patient in the hospital.

I was in for ten days, during which time it became clear that I would need some sort of operation to fix what Harrison thought was the cause of my problems. The accident had given rise to a good deal of scarring throughout my biliary system. As a result, ducts through which my digestive juices flowed from the liver and the pancreas were narrowed. This caused a sludgy backup to clog my system, and it eventually backed right up into the pancreas. The result: catastrophe. The solution was to cut a larger opening at the ampulla, the vessel through which all these juices flowed into my stomach. The operation had to wait till the acute phase of my condition had passed; my hospital stay was therefore meant to be restorative.

After a week or so, two roommates from my days at Queen's—both named John (let's call them One and Two)—turned up for a visit on a Sunday afternoon, and we snuck out to see a movie. I felt like a character from *One Flew Over the Cuckoo's Nest*, AWOL from the pervasive atmosphere of illness. For one afternoon we were breaking away from the hospital's authority and the unconscious discipline of recovery. Both Johns are well over six feet three inches tall. Walking along between them, I felt myself disappear. Soon enough the recklessness that is the lifeblood of male friendship took hold, and we were teasing and shouting like a pack of hyenas, slinging arm punches followed by whoops and cackles and the inevitable reprisals. Even in my enfeebled state I was engaging in the usual give-and-take. At one stage I even bounced a shot off John One's shoulder, which was duly repaid. Still, I was fidgety and nervous in their presence. Both of them were already terribly accomplished in their fields, John One as an executive in the toy business and John

Two as a diplomat working for the United Nations. I had the same sensation I'd had as a teenager: humiliated by my physical diminution and fragility at the same time as I was willing, even relieved, to be the subject of another's pity and protectiveness. Strange.

The afternoon ended when they deposited me back in my bed. They had about them the air of men who'd done a good and not altogether unpleasant deed. They waved and then shuffled their large frames out through the door. I lay on the bed with my socked feet crossed, my arms folded across my chest, and drifted off into a contented sleep. I remember thinking, as I dropped away, that it was the first time in ages that I'd felt the relaxed, snoozy sensation of a normal Sunday afternoon.

I was sent home in the middle of the following week. My primary concern wasn't so much whether I should go back to work immediately but at what point other people would think me lax for failing to turn up. For the most part, surgeons and surgical residents take a rather Old Testament view of recovery. "You'll get back to yourself as fast as you *will* yourself to do so. A professional who is concerned and energized by his work will be back at it in the shortest time possible. An unmotivated, unemployed guy will sit around on his can either way." Probably true, but thank God they didn't take to the psychiatric portion of the intern's rotation.

I was at home for about ten days, during which time I sat out on the back porch rereading *On the Road*. For the first time I thought that my own recent adventures might make a hell of a story, with Jean as Florence Nightingale cum Dean Moriarty and me as a sort of intubated Sal Paradise. What is it about that book? So much adolescent, restless, uninhibited behaviour—every page is soaked in it. The characters are full of energy, engaging everything for its own sake, a sensibility utterly at odds with my own:

> He dragged his long thin body around the entire United States and most of Europe and North Africa in his time, only to see what was going on; he married a white Russian countess in Yugoslavia to get her away from the Nazis in the thirties; there are pictures of him with the international cocaine set of the thirties—gangs with white hair, leaning on one another; there are other pictures of him in a Panama hat, surveying the streets of Algiers: he never saw the white Russian countess again. He was an exterminator in Chicago, a bartender in New York, a summons-server in Newark. In Paris he sat at café tables, watching the sullen French faces go by. In Athens he looked up from his ouzo at what he called the ugliest people in the world. In Istanbul he threaded his way through crowds of opium addicts and rug-sellers, looking for the facts. In English hotels he read Spengler and the Marquis de Sade. In Chicago he planned to hold up a Turkish bath, hesitated just for two minutes too long for a drink, and wound up with two dollars and had had to make a run for it. He did all these things merely for experience.

I, on the other hand, sat on the back porch of my house in downtown Toronto drinking coffee and waiting for my mother to turn up most mornings with five newspapers, which I ploughed through in anxious anticipation of having to start my new job at the *Globe*. The editor seemed non-plussed at my absence. When I finally arrived for my first day on the job, four weeks behind schedule, he made a big deal of telling me not to feel as though I had to rush back.

In the event, the job was a disaster. The economy was in free fall, and the supplement was losing a ton of money. The editor was a square-headed man who wore a pair of chunky Politburo-style glasses. I always pictured him in a heavy overcoat, waving to the masses from the top of Lenin's tomb while a large Soviet military parade marched by.

Looking to hedge his bets, the editor hired another underling, the former staff editor from the business magazine. My boss did everything to me but hold up a sign reading "Get the fuck out." I failed to pick up even a whiff of what was to come.

On the day I was to go for surgery, he called me into his office and fired me. Of course I've played the whole thing over and over in my mind—how I stand up and confront him. In truth I got a lump in my throat, imagined it was all my fault and thanked him for not firing me sooner. Gutsy.

I clambered into a cab and made my way up to Sunnybrook. It was a cold, concrete-grey day. The wind pushed the leaves around the crescent driveway, and I mounted the steps to the entry hall with a growing sense of foreboding. I was scheduled for day surgery with a Dr. Cohen, whom I'd met for about ten seconds two months earlier, during the last few days of my previous stay. I was prepped in an upstairs holding area—stripped of my clothes and dressed in one of those backless hospital gowns designed to make the patient feel like a supplicant, exposed and vulnerable—before being taken down on a gurney to a sort of combination X-ray/operating room in the basement.

Left alone outside the O.R., I closed my eyes and tried to fight off the irrational fears that breed like flies in any empty hospital corridor. When I opened my eyes, there at the end of the gurney, wearing one of those green surgical caps that might be confused with the white ones they wear at a slaughterhouse, was Dr. Cohen. For some reason I felt it important that he know I'd just been fired from my job at *The Globe and Mail*, as though even getting fired by that organization was an august occasion.

Cohen said something jokey and sympathetic, and then things began to move quickly. I was rolled into the room. There seemed to be a lot of nurses standing around, and I felt all their hands working me into a suitable position, prone on the table, my ass in the air so that I felt whatever breeze was wafting in the room move over my privates. Seconds later I was getting a shot of Valium intravenously. I remember thinking that some sort of creamy custard was being poured into my veins, and soon the very essence of me was a flowing custard, slow and rich and thick. As I felt this sensation ooze through me, I heard Cohen joking with the nurses. "Can anybody here get this guy a job? . . . He's a journalist. There must be a lot of jobs around for a guy like that."

I joined in the general merriment at my predicament, fired from my job one minute and the next propped up on a table like a prize roast pig. The operation itself consisted of Cohen shoving a length of rubber tubing down my throat. Attached to the end of the tube were various tiny scalpels, pincers and a camera. The level of consciousness at which I was maintained allowed Cohen to order up whatever flex or movement he required in order to better carve or grasp whatever it was he sought to slice or retrieve. Turned away from me, staring at a screen off to one side, he would command distractedly, "Push up your diaphragm. A little more. That's it." Though the sensation delivered by the Valium wasn't wholly unpleasant, dulling the pain and the indignity of the procedure, there was occasionally a sharp twinge deep inside to remind me that I was being cut open from the inside out.

Later, in the recovery room, as I climbed the stairs of perception, that twinge grew more prominent. Jean came to pick me up, and as I made my slow, wobbly way to the car, the pain began to rise up and I could make out the shark again. We didn't get even halfway home before we turned around and headed back to Emergency. I was given a shot. Cohen turned up looking unhappily perplexed, as though I were his brand new lawn mower gone immediately on the fritz.

It was a busy night. While waiting to be moved onto a ward, I lay double-parked in a gurney with an older woman beside me, who moaned repeatedly through an oxygen mask, "Do they know I'm here? They do, don't they? Know (gasp) I'm (gasp) here."

My father turned up. "Poor old sod," he said, patting me on the leg. This made me feel so much better that if I'd had more energy I would have shed a tear.

Later, Jean told me a story about my father going to phone my mum to let her know everything was more or less in order. Jean spied him standing in front of a pay phone at the end of the hall, and even at a distance she could see that he was perplexed. "Now," he asked as she approached, speaking in his slow, measured cadence. "How . . . does . . . this . . . go?" Jean told this story to me with a mixture of astonishment and admiration. "You know, I'm quite certain he hadn't used a pay phone in twenty-five years."

The next day I felt better. I sat cross-legged on the bed while Cohen held forth before a band of residents and interns. A teaching hospital, while providing far and away the best care to patients with complex conditions, also turns the patient into the subject of the doctors' practical and intellectual curiosity. The band of doctors stood in a semi-circle at the end of the bed as I tried to look bright-eyed and bushy-tailed. It seemed I had suffered a bout of pancreatitis brought on by the surgery itself.

My starkest sensation that morning was of the distance between the doctors and the person sitting on the bed. I was reminded of engineering students at Queen's staring at equations on a blackboard, their eyes blank as their minds worked at a level of abstraction much higher than I could imagine. I hoped that whatever the doctor tried, it would take hold, since I suspected that if it did not, I would evolve into a problem more to be puzzled over than solved.

As it turned out, the next few weeks were difficult. I remember one conversation in particular, with my mother, in which she told me that my cousin Geoff's stag had carried on without me, clearly at her behest. It hit me all at once: I was turning thirty, I'd lost the one job I thought would finally put me clear of my mother's skepticism concerning my prospects, and I found myself once again the victim of her maternal fierceness. As I screamed myself hoarse over the phone, I could hear the tones of her voice in my own as though she were inhabiting me. I couldn't tell exactly who it was I was shouting at, mother or myself. Nevertheless, I continued to scream into the phone even as I heard the dial tone emerge after her end of the line went dead.

By the spring of the following year, things had turned around a bit. I had gone to Poland, where I'd reported a story for *Saturday Night* magazine. The opportunity to travel as a "foreign correspondent" had lightened my mood considerably. At the same time, I was anxious at having to write a story chronicling the exploits of the young American and Canadian economists who were directing Poland towards a free market economy after the fall of the Berlin Wall.

Journalism was a way into writing without commitment. You could lose yourself in the imperatives of others. The fear of pretention, the fear of ostentation, the fear that someone might turn to you at some point and, appraising everything about you in a single moment, say, "And who do you think *you* are?"—all that was neatly addressed by journalism's relentless espousal of the writer's anonymity.

My mother had managed to get her oar in the water by persuading me to take cartons and cartons of dried low-fat soups, which she insisted I eat at every occasion. According to mum, the Poles' entire diet consisted of lard. I still remember the quizzical look on the face of a Polish customs officer as he pulled the cartons out of my bag while I explained in loud, slow colonial English that "I had rather a bad accident as a teenager that resulted in my acquiring pancreatitis."

"Huh?"

"Look, it's a disease of the stomach," I said, pulling up my shirt to show the bureaucrat my scars.

The cartons sat unused in a corner of my Polish hotel room, as they would in the corners of other hotel rooms throughout eastern Europe as I travelled various precincts during the first half of the 1990s, my mother's admonitions ringing in my (deafened) ears.

On my return from Poland in February 1991, I received a call concerning the health of my friend Marcus's wife, Jacqui. The previous winter I had visited her in the hospital, where she'd had some sort of operation for cancer. Jacqui was a bright, aggressive lawyer, an avowed feminist, who could be salty and tart, and I liked that. She'd sat cross-legged on the bed, her upturned nose seeming to pull up the rest of her face in a smile. The conversation had been jokey and warm. We'd traded war stories about nurses and doctors like a couple of aging vaudevillians.

I'd lost contact with Marcus and Jacqui over the course of the last year, what with my own health and career crises, and now Jacqui had taken a turn for the worse. As the disease took hold, she and Marcus were married in a quiet private ceremony. By the time I got the call in February from one of her oldest friends, Jacqui was, in effect, receiving palliative care at Toronto General. The friend broached the idea of organizing a group of us to work in shifts around the clock, so that Jacqui wouldn't be alone. I signed up. In addition, I made calls to the old gang from Queen's. At one time or another over those several weeks before her death, everybody showed up either to visit or to work. I sensed an air of caution and contrition about us, as though we had all committed the same unnamed sin and were seeking the possibility of remission through good works.

As for Marcus, and Jacqui's family, their grief seemed to me opaque and beyond understanding. I remember Marcus telling me that a CAT scan of Jacqui's brain had revealed so many tumours—white dots against the brain's dark background—that it looked like a snowstorm in her skull. One night, sitting on a counter in a supply room, his large feet dangling above the floor, Marcus told me that his wife was dying and he couldn't understand why. His voice cracked like a gunshot on the word *why*, and the tears flew out of him like raindrops bouncing off a windshield.

One day I turned up at the hospital having written that day's lead story in *The Globe and Mail* sports section, an odd piece about a stumpy Soviet hockey coach who'd come from Belarus to head up the hockey program at Trinity College School in Port Hope, Ontario. When I came into the room, filled with her friends and family, Jacqui, whose eroding facial features confirmed her body's betrayal, worked up a warm smile and announced, "It's our friend the writer," and she asked me to autograph the article. In the midst of the sustained horror that the remainder of her life had become, Jacqui took care to make me feel good about *my*self. Later, she said simply that she hoped I would keep at my writing, that I seemed to have a talent for it; I wasn't to waste it or get sidetracked. If there's an absolute proof that context is everything, this was it.

Still, I failed to recognize the real lesson of Jacqui's mortality. In the end she died and I didn't, and somehow I had to find the sense in that, just as I'd had to make sense of the little girl's death when I was laid up after my accident. In my head, the girl's death hadn't really been her death at all, but another crucible through which I passed in overcoming adversity. Jacqui too was a means: "My death will make you stronger." I couldn't put myself in her place, and of course this is all wrong. In death there is nothing but the end. It's not about me. In a way it's not about the person who is dying, either. It's about death. The little child clutching his mother as the plane goes down. Go there. Try it. Die a little. You might as well—you're going there anyway.

When we really love somebody, I mean *really* love somebody—when even for a second we forget about who we are and how this is affecting *me*—we die a little too, because it's not about us, it's about them; and when it's like that you might as well be falling off a cliff, you're that vulnerable.

A couple of months later, at Jacqui's funeral, I stood in a sort of raggle-taggle receiving line as Marcus made his way into the church. He looked shrunken and defeated in a jacket and tie, his neck insufficient to meet the purpose of his collar. I stuck out my right hand to shake his. On his left, a woman fell tearfully into his arm. As he held her, his right mitt was stuck in mine. For some reason I decided to give him a two-hander, as though one more hand might somehow buck him up. He looked at me, then down at my double-hand clutch. He chuckled slightly, as if gently to admonish me. I released his hand.

Later, we gathered at a friend's house and none of us said anything that mattered. The light that day seemed pale and inconsequential, as though the sun were rushing embarrassed across the sky.

A NORMAL LIFE

We are not cold, poor, hungry, lonely, or miserable in any other common way, so why should so many of us struggle to forget our happy lot? Is it the ineradicable strain of guilt and vengefulness in man's nature?

—JOHN CHEEVER, *The Journals of John Cheever*

OVER THE NEXT SEVERAL YEARS my health held steady. Cohen's operation seemed to have done the trick. I found it hard in some ways to give up the sense of self that my illness had engendered in me. Though I still tended to dine out on my troubles, I did so more and more self-consciously, as if my good health were putting the lie to my heroic self. Or was it that the ill health excused my indolence and sloppy behaviour?

In June 1992, Jean gave birth to our first child, Charlotte. During the birth I became very agitated at what I thought was the medical staff's languid pace in relieving my wife's pain. When the anaesthetist finally arrived, I was in a rage. I see now that I wasn't treating the birth of our first child as a glorious event in our lives, but as a painful medical condition that needed relief.

My state was hardly relieved by the doctor's oily manner and appearance. He had slick hair and one of those thin moustaches that bisects an otherwise clean-shaven upper lip *à la* John Waters. He referred to Jean as "princess." I was "hubby." As he prepared to insert the epidural needle into Jean's spine, he asked that I hold her by the shoulders so as to ensure that she not fall over or otherwise interrupt the needle's smooth entry. The needle entering the spinal column sounded like a dead branch snapping off a tree, and in a moment my past was all over me. I felt myself stagger backwards as I slipped slowly down the wall, glancing my noggin off the sink on the way down. While falling I heard the doctor, oozing calm, say to no one in particular, "Oops, hubby doesn't look so good."

Just after midnight, having watched the birth of my first child and recovered my senses, I walked Charlotte around the birthing theatre. We stopped by a window on the hospital's south side and watched the highway's streaming traffic and the lights of the city beyond.

Parenting was something I confess I gave up on almost before I'd started. Actually, I didn't give up on it so much as I kept imagining I could put it off, as though it were a bill I should probably pay or a return luncheon date I needed to honour. At the same time it was a perfect excuse for putting off everything and everyone else. "I can't go out, I can't do anything . . . I have kids." The problem, of course, is that you can't put kids off. Not parenting isn't like procrastinating. It's more like you're waiting for somebody else to break the glass on that emergency box, the one that signals Children's Aid that your kids require immediate intervention.

Charlotte fell victim to my lassitude/anxiety dialectic more than once. I remember trying to build the crib that would keep her safe the first several years of life. I sat around for hours contemplating the work required—doing nothing, just contemplating. Then the sun dropped and the baby needed to go to bed—preferably not our bed. Immediately, I began to panic, and in a moment I was a whirlwind of uncoordinated activity. Shoving here, wrenching there, the pieces of the puzzle refused to line up in such a way as to spell *crib*. Then my thumb got jammed amidst the workings of a mechanism that slides up and down, and I found myself screaming, trying to remove my thumb and with each tug feeling a more and more acute crushing sensation. A moment later, somehow, my thumb was free and I was incredibly angry . . . at . . . at . . . them. I stared daggers at the source of my pain. My wife and child stood at the door to the small room, my daughter crying and reaching for me. And I realized that, like it or not, I *was* parenting. Running around like an idiot, screaming and cursing the eternal souls of your wife and progeny, is as formative of character as a kind word and a gently cupped chin. It's a matter of choice.

Once the contraption was functioning more or less like a crib, we decided we were booting Charlotte out of our bed permanently. We even had a method: Ferberizing, named for a certain Dr. Ferber, whose book essentially advocated turning a blind eye and deaf ear to the child's tortured yearning for comfort, except for the occasional reassuring word doled out at intervals. Oh yeah, and you were supposed to put up a chart recording the number of times you visited the child's room each night—never, of course, having any physical contact of any kind. This we did. Night after living night.

Oftentimes we failed and brought Charlotte into our bed, snuffling and quivering with rage at the indignity of her suffering. In the world of the good Dr. Ferber this was clearly a failure of will on our part, and we were suitably guilt-ridden.

One night, in the midst of a particularly brutal session ("you go" . . . "no you go" . . . "no, fuck, you go"), Jean and I were lying in bed listening to Charlotte belt out the primordial misery of the disconsolate child. Suddenly, she stopped. The air was soaked in silence. Jean and I looked at each other with a mixture of hope and trepidation. Then, in a basso profundo, strangely calm voice that seemed to emanate from another being entirely, we heard "Help."

I was out of the bed and down the hall in a shot. From the doorway I saw that Charlotte had flipped herself over the railing and was now hanging by one arm, which was caught between the slats of the crib. She looked up at me, her face neither fearful nor expectant. And again, "Help." I scooped her up as Jean came running in behind me. We buried our faces in our daughter as though our fevered kisses were an act of penance. That was the last of Dr. Ferber.

During this time mum was constantly on the scene, and as I look back now, I'm grateful for her presence. At the time, though, I was a good deal less sanguine. She always seemed to remind me of what it was I was trying to get away from. But my usual complaints started sounding dissonant to my own ear. Children are permanent. The things they need, fundamentally, do not change from one generation to the next: order, discipline and consistency. It's not mysterious. And yet, in my arrogant, self-involved fashion, I imagined that my shortcomings were conscious acts of division—

ways of separating my child from what had come before. And though I see it for what it is now, then I just thought my mother was a meddling biddy with too much time on her hands. Imagine the temerity: cleaning the house, tending the garden, having our sofa recovered, waxing the dining-room table, polishing the silver, mending the curtain.

During this period mum was on the whole coming to terms with her life. She'd stopped drinking quite so much. I think on the whole she slept better. I remember during the bad patches, the long, sleepless nights fuelled by gin—which somehow kept my mother up—she used to move the furniture repeatedly around the drawing room. The next morning our nearsighted schnauzer would peel out from the kitchen heading for the greenhouse door, with predictable results.

Mum reconciled herself, in whatever way middle-aged people do, to the blunt fact of her marriage. In her case this meant deciding that her life was her own and that she had to find her own way. She travelled a lot in search of the things that could be backgrounds against which her life might reveal itself. In the journal I kept for a while after mum first announced she was dying, there is this entry: "Later she talked about somebody called Ernesto, whose apartment she had visited along the Grand canal. Mum's eyes narrowed and widened theatrically as she described the walls of that apartment, a mix of plaster and marble dust that gave off a brilliant sheen."

Looking back, I wish I'd found the pith in that. Instead, I was for the most part suspicious and prickly. It seemed I could never just appreciate her as a woman growing graciously into her elderly self. I was a boy failing to recognize the possibility of his own redemption or his mother's. *How dare she get old and frail and feisty in the face of time? I haven't finished growing up, dammit. I'm still lazy and careless and I don't know what I want. Who's going to pick me up after school? Who's going to answer for my failings? Who?*

I still don't know.

I suppose if there was one thing I took genuine pleasure in as mum aged, it was her speech. Beyond the parochial idiosyncrasies of class, my mother had a rich, varied, slightly eccentric command of the English language.

An argument was never just an argument, it was "a real donnybrook." Peculiar behaviour proved that the person in question was "as mad as a hatter." One never simply broke something, one "smashed it to smithereens." People weren't just in high spirits, "they carried on like the Tiller girls." Things weren't just big, they were "ginormous." (I actually tried to sneak the word *ginormous* past the editors of *Canadian Business* magazine. A working-class Brit rebuffed me, saying that the pages of his magazine weren't the place for "Rosedale idiosyncrasies.")

If you had time on your hands, you were "as free as the breeze in the trees." Good news was "jolly hockey sticks." Anything my mother couldn't name was a thingamajig. Anyone she couldn't name was Mr. or Mrs. Thingummy. Goodbye was never just goodbye, it was "I'll have to love you and leave you." You didn't just sleep well, you "slept like a frog on a log." Naughty behaviour tinged with wit or cleverness was greeted with "You'll come to a bad end, ma' boy." Trouble meant you were in a "sticky wicket." Mum never asked simply that a light be turned on to fend off the increasing gloom; it was "Could we perhaps shed a little light on the subject?"

Her phone manner was equally fascinating. Whereas the vast majority of us answer the phone with "Hello," mum insisted on "Yeeessss?" This was delivered as a faintly aggressive interrogative, as in "Do you have anything interesting to say to me? If so—out with it."

Ever since mum died, any time I hear one of these expressions, whether in passing or deep in conversation, I have the same electrified feeling. It's as though the former love of my life has just walked into the room after an extended absence.

In the spring of 1996 our second child, Anne, was born. Mum had just announced that she was dying of cancer. Once again I ran afoul of the medical practitioners. Jean had gone over term and was scheduled to be induced. After having her water broken to no effect, it was decided to proceed with a dose of Pitocin, which tricks the body into producing contractions. The difficulty is that induced contractions tend to come at irregular intervals, which makes the pain that much harder to bear. Jean's natural stoicism and control broke down in the face of this, and I found myself angrily demanding that something be done to ease her pain.

The nurse on hand was full to the brim with folk wisdom. "You must be patient, Mr. Bell, it's really up to Mother Nature and Father Time."

"I don't really care for your home truths," I replied. "I want you to do something for my wife's pain, and I want you to do it now. And if you can't, perhaps I'll find someone who will."

The nurse more or less fled the scene.

Eventually, Jean's pain was sorted out thanks to another

epidural. Looking back at an entry in my journal of that time, I find myself oddly comparing my efforts to retain a sense of detached cool in the face of Jean's difficult labour with my attempts to stay calm in the face of my mother's sometimes bitter conversation. "On both occasions I feel my hold on the right way/good form growing tenuous."

MOTHER

We rise from sleep all natural men, boisterous, loving, and hopeful, but the dark faced stranger is waiting at the door, the viper is coiled in the garden . . .

—JOHN CHEEVER, *The Journals of John Cheever*

IN THE LATE SUMMER OF 1996, my mother started on a form of oral chemotherapy. The open wounds that signalled the spread of the cancer from her chest wall into her arm healed up, and she was able to venture out of bed for the first time in months. As she did so, I imagined that she would recover. Dad seemed optimistic too, and in my mind's eye I pictured her at the cottage swimming through her cancer the way she'd swum along the shore at Lake Simcoe, doing her stately breaststroke, heart thudding away inside her chest, head never ducking under the waterline, hair enclosed in one of those fancy rubber skullcaps you might see in an Esther Williams movie.

Over the next couple of years, following Anne's birth and during the Indian summer of my mother's cancer, I fell into my work. I pursued every opportunity that came my way—television, radio, editing *Shift* magazine, freelancing as a third-string movie reviewer and entertainment writer for *The Globe and Mail.* I lived on adrenalin and rage. I rehearsed the violent deaths of friends, relatives, acquaintances, colleagues, anyone who for any reason I felt had slighted me. It didn't take much. One night Jean had to physically restrain me from charging down to *The Globe and Mail* to beat up the then arts editors. I imagined the satisfying sound of their knees splintering under mighty blows from my aluminum baseball bat. I can't recall the nature of the slight. I do remember a look in Jean's eye that suggested that even by my standards my behaviour was way beyond the pale.

Just before Christmas 1997, dad contracted a horrible case of pneumonia and was hospitalized at Sunnybrook. Mum was failing, so it fell to me to keep a sharp lookout on his condition. Dad was very weak and he'd had a tube stuck into his chest. His hair was greasy and dishevelled, his face unshaven. These in themselves were dramatic deviations from the military norm.

I was wandering out of the hospital, utterly distressed, when I caught myself and remembered to query the nursing staff. Though things were far from ideal, I figured two things were in dad's corner: the nurses obviously knew who he was, and they went on about how much worse he'd been only a day earlier. I called mum at home from an empty dialysis clinic, propped up in one of the dentist-style chairs in which, during the day, patients get their blood washed. The first words out of mum's mouth were, "Well, we'll just have to sell the house. I can't reasonably nurse your father back to health carting his meals up and down stairs." I heard in her tone the brittle, near-hysterical quality that always raised my ire. I leaped to the conclusion that mum was going to sell the house out from under dad's nose from some delayed form of marital spite.

But what followed over the next ten months or so was a gavotte of love, duty and devotion between my parents that even now leaves me breathless. It challenged all my preconceptions, and to this day I am confused and disquieted at the degree to which I underestimated the resources and rectitude of both my mother and my father.

My mum moved quickly to buy a condominium apartment in a building at the corner of Jarvis and Carlton. It struck me as an odd location in which to buy. It's around the corner from the city's gay ghetto—epicentre of the annual Gay Pride Parade—and sits across the street from a park well known as a sanctuary for the homeless and addled. But as the months went by, I began to see the genius of my mother's instincts; how her decision was based on a more sophisticated calculus than even the propriety with which she'd raised me. Mum's Potemkin protests concerning the impossibility of caring for dad while he recovered from his pneumonia masked a more profound concern—that running a household on three floors without the support of staff would be too much strain for dad once he started caring for her as she succumbed to the cancer. Mum anticipated that dad would pursue his duty to care for her to the last with an ardour and devotion in keeping with his natural instincts. She wanted to give him the space to live up to her expectations.

In March 1998, dad called to say that mum and my aunt Janet would be going down to the new apartment to inspect the renovations. It was clear by this time that the oral chemo had run its course and the cancer was back with a vengeance in mum's left arm. When I came to the door, she appeared, listing to her left with a large pillow jammed between her arm and her chest. She was ghastly pale but looked ready for a fight, her eyes glinting and jaw set. My mother's relationship with the next oldest Ambridge girl was complicated by the sense that her authority and status as the eldest was in some way threatened by Janet's having married into money more substantial even than my father's. Mum believed she was the more accomplished of the two, and yet money brings its own authority.

The battle lines were clearly drawn. Mum was preparing to justify her decision to uproot after fifteen years and move to an area her sister would sniff at. I took her arm in mine and helped her into Janet's car. For the first time I encountered the tremble and terrible wasting of the disease. When we got to the apartment, I felt myself standing apart from the scene as my mother and Janet played out the strategic engagement of a long-standing sibling rivalry.

Mum fired off her carefully prepared anecdotal rounds: a bank president lived in the building and refused the bank's efforts to relocate him into more glamorous digs; a lifelong friend of my parents, Robert Macauley (the leading intellectual of his generation in Ontario politics), was a fellow tenant and was trotted out as the chief advocate for my mother's decision. Janet showed admirable restraint under this barrage, but I must admit I enjoyed watching mum aggressively taking charge. It was a clear late winter day, and as we made our way around the bare concrete floors, the sun steamed through the place, warming my face. The view from the eleventh floor past the city's skyscrapers and church steeples all the way down to the lakefront was spectacular.

As I helped mum back into the car, she turned to me and asked in a thoroughly mischievous tone if I would please go and get her some cigarettes. Suddenly, the smug distance I'd maintained was gone, though I tried to play the cool Sardonios. Mum was having none of it. "Don't be difficult, just get on with it," she said. I moved sheepishly across the street and into a convenience store, where I bought a pack of Craven "A" filters. As I did so, I accepted that her life included smoking cigarettes and would continue to do so in the face of her mortality. I walked back to the car, handed her the fags and looked away as she lit up and took in that first relieved breath, the smoke flowing smoothly down into her lungs and up and out through her mouth and nose.

In late May 1998, I began to make preparations for a trip to Buenos Aires. I was so excited I could have spit. I would be there during the World Cup and would be interviewing the left-wing poet, essayist and intellectual Eduardo Galeano. The week before, mother had called me at the office, prefacing her remarks by stating that she was so angry she could barely speak.

"Do you ever think of anyone other than yourself? Have you even bothered to get your medical records translated into Spanish?"

"Of course I have," I fibbed.

I then went on to describe in rather too vivid detail the arrangements I'd made to ensure my safety. I invented a fabulous network of friends and important contacts awaiting me as though I were a head of state. Mother's anger dissipated only slightly. Why couldn't I think of my children or the sacrifices that Jean made on my behalf? she prodded. I found myself laughing, half in disbelief, at her accusations. "Mother, for Christ's sakes, what's bothering you? It can't be this. What's this all about?" This only served to swell her titanic rage.

In fact I knew perfectly well what this was all about. My mother's illness allowed her no recourse. If things were going to go wrong for me, there wasn't a thing she could do about it; she could afford me no protection. She had only her death left to contemplate.

When I got back from Argentina, I went to see her straight away. She questioned me closely regarding the architecture, art, politics and manners of the place. I did my best to answer. I told her about going to meet with Galeano in Montevideo. I was very animated in this discussion, though I can't remember the exact cut and thrust.

Every detail of my encounter with Galeano had thrilled me. On a fax to me, his signature was illustrated with a stylized stick figure of a pig. What could that mean? Then another fax: "I'll be waiting at the café on Friday 19 2:30 PM—a little earlier than the hour I told you, because of the match Spain Paraguay, which begins at 4. Yours, Eduardo." *Yours, Eduardo*. And again the pig figure.

Over the next couple of days, between appointments for other stories, I wandered the claustrophobic streets of downtown Buenos Aires, reading a book of Galeano's collected journalism, *We Say No*. Late in the evening, chowing down on superb Argentine beef and red wine, I found myself moved to tears by the sheer emotional weight Galeano lays on the reader. Of course it was mostly the wine and partly being alone among fourteen million people, but there is something cinematic about Galeano's prose. It passes stealthily through your rational self and takes hold of you somewhere further down the spinal column.

> I read my mother a sample:
> To claim that literature on its own is going to change reality is an act of madness or arrogance. It seems to me no less foolish to deny that it can aid in making this change. The awareness of our limitations is undoubtedly an awareness of our reality. Amid the fog of desperation and doubt, it is possible to face it and wrestle with it—with our limitations, but at the same time in opposition to them . . . Our effectiveness depends on our capacity to be audacious and astute, clear and appealing. I would hope that we can create a language more fearless and beautiful than that used by conformist writers to greet the twilight.

There is something both clear-eyed and romantic about this notion. Galeano is constantly balancing his readers on a knife's edge between rushing to the clarion call of the great cause and stopping short as he skewers some received truth or other.

> I don't share the attitude of those who demand special freedom for writers, independently of freedom for other workers. Great changes, deep structural changes, will be necessary in our countries if we writers are to go beyond the citadels of the elites, if we are to express ourselves, free of visible and invisible restraints. In an incarcerated society, free literature can exist only as denunciation and hope.

I noticed mum was taking notes as I ran off at the mouth. What, I wondered, does she make of her son, the well-born commie sympathizer?

Less than a week after my return from Argentina I went away again for a month, to the Banff Centre for the Arts to write a piece on the summer of my accident. I began to realize then that my experience of mother's illness was now as much a part of my accident as the ripples washing across a pond are the result of the splash from a stone. I couldn't make out the breadth or even the shape of this truth at that time. I wrote in a fishing boat that had been adapted as a writer's studio on the side of a mountain in Alberta and I phoned mum at moments when I felt triumphant because at those times there didn't seem to be anyone else in the world I wanted to talk to. Our conversations were gossipy and full of laughs. One day I made so much noise hooting at my mother's wisecracks that another writer in the colony walked up from his cabin and slammed my door.

I wilfully ignored the failing timbre of her voice and the dulling of her manner. I sat in my boat, tapping on the keyboard, while Sarah McLachlan sang in my ear. (As I wrote that summer, I developed a dreadful habit. To test the sad bits, I would write and rewrite them while playing melancholy music on my Walkman—the more blubbering and sentimental, the better.)

By the time I was home again, my mother was finally and irrevocably on her way. Dad was doing a superb job nursing her. I wasn't sure of my role except to show up, which I did three days a week through August and September. Each time was difficult in its way. After each visit I wandered out onto Carlton Street, the early evening light growing dimmer by the day, and then through the old CBC studios just north of Carlton or around the greenhouses in Allan Gardens. After a visit I'd sometimes call a friend or acquaintance out of the blue and carry on a sad, distracted conversation. I wandered around my life like a deep-sea diver poking around on the sea floor, my vision strangely truncated, my responses slow and awkward.

One day near the end I dropped over in the early afternoon. I was apprehensive more about seeing dad than mum. I'd been coming over later and later in the evenings, using my job as an excuse. The previous night my father had suddenly turned on me as I came through the door.

"How old are you?" he had asked.

I felt my bile rise. "Do you want me to make a schedule, is that it?"

"It's too late for her to be seeing anybody."

Suddenly I flashed to my teenage self in the kitchen of our house on Lonsdale. I was slicing roast beef for a late evening snack. Dad came into the kitchen and gave me a dirty look for no reason I knew of. Suddenly, just like that, I was pointing the knife at him. "Have you got a problem with this?" I asked him. "What the fuck are you gonna do about it? What are you going to do?" Dad's eyes grew wide and he beat a retreat from his son the psychopath.

Now, in the afternoon, I went through to see mum in her room, taking my usual spot at the end of the bed. She seemed both tetchy and distant. I put this down to the painkillers. She began to discuss in a rather abstract way a book that she claimed her sister Shirley was planning to write. This news seemed to annoy her. I prodded to find out more. Mum waved her good hand in a vague motion to indicate it was neither here nor there.

Shirley lived in Colorado and had recently come down with a rather serious case of Parkinson's disease. It was likely the whole notion of a book was the product of a drug-induced misapprehension of my mother's. Still, what was Shirley doing writing a book? I mean, what qualifications did Shirley have to be writing a book? At least I had a track record. I mean, did she even have a publisher? I'd like to report that I had the good sense to keep a consoling look about my face as my inner self churned away with all this claptrap; but no, every word of it escaped my lips.

At the conclusion of this self-indulgent aria I noticed mother scowling at me over her reading glasses.

"What?"

"Don't," she said, having come all the way back to herself, "be so pompous." She paused then, like Muhammad Ali watching George Foreman tumbling towards the canvas that steamy night in Kinshasa, Zaire. Unlike Ali, my mother couldn't resist pasting me on the way down. "Just," she added, the leather thudding behind my ear, "like your father."

And the thing is, she was right, and I thought of her heart pounding away and for a moment I wondered, how can she die? How can somebody see right through you one minute and be gone the next? But that wasn't the real question. The real question was why couldn't I talk to her about her death and dying, reach out and touch the part of her she had saved in me?

Soon enough I began to see just how it was she could die, how her strength could be sapped by the drugs and the disease, how her body and mind could collapse around her soul.

One afternoon she pointed to an aqua blue perfume bottle. I'd seen it so many times before that I'd stopped registering its existence. It was beautiful nonetheless. In a fading voice mum told me her version of how it came into her possession. "It's French, nineteenth-century, I think. It was brought back to me from Europe by a little girl named Bev

Wood. We were living in St. Catharines at the time." Mum paused, then spoke again. "She wasn't even my best friend."

There was in that a tone I'd rarely, if ever, heard from her. She was mystified. *Why would Bev Wood have given me that precious object? Why?*

There were innumerable mysteries in my mother's life, as there are in every life, and they would die with her. Was I one of those mysteries? Or was it me that was mystified, raised in privilege in a world where there weren't meant to be any questions left to answer, where the certainty of comfort and position was all and destiny simply a matter of picking up one's ordained legacy and carrying it?

October 1, 1998, was grey and cool, full of flat light, the first day that indicated fall was on the way. I went to see her as usual. Dad caught me at the door. "Watch her, will you?" he asked.

I sat with my mother for a long time. At first she was in an almost playful mood. Dad brought her lunch and gave her a gentle ribbing. She picked up her glass of wine: "Pour this on his head, will you?" Later, though, her mind started to wander aimlessly, and her complexion turned ominously dark, somewhere between puce and brown. Was it her or the light in the room? Mum started talking about an opera and got confused as to whether or not Joan Sutherland had appeared.

Moments later her old friend Rita Temelkof arrived. Mum and Rita had always shared a certain *vieux monde* snobbery as they talked about paintings and opera and ballet, and the philistine in me rose up the back of my throat whenever Rita turned up. She sat down in my place as soon as I got up to go. As I left, I heard mum making the same point about the opera and once again confusing herself. "Was Joan Sutherland in the damn thing or not?"

I spoke to dad for a while before heading to the elevator. Just as I stepped on, I saw Rita leave the apartment with her shoulders slumped and her head drooped forward. I hopped on the elevator and wished it would hurry on down to the ground.

During the last week of my mother's life she was sweet and solicitous almost to a fault. Her behaviour seemed somehow climactic. Partway through one visit, dad interrupted to say that her palliative care physician, Dr. Colette Hegarty, had arrived. I thought I should be going, but dad held me up just outside the bedroom door. The situation was getting desperate. He was exhausted. Despite her brave show for me, my mother's pain demanded the meds be renewed at a pace requiring constant medical supervision. If her situation deteriorated, she would have to be moved to the palliative care unit at the Salvation Army Hospital, where Dr. Hegarty was on staff.

Dad presented all this matter-of-factly. I decided to live in hope. Maybe, I thought in the face of a terminal cancer that was chewing her to bits, she'll get better.

While Dr. Hegarty and mum discussed the road to the hereafter, I sat and stared at the oversized illustrated titles in my parents' library: *Irish Glass*, *19th Century Glass*, *Filosofiana: The Villa of Piazza Armerina*. I picked up a large leather-bound tome, *The Complete Dictionary of Arts and Science*, that had belonged to my grandfather Ambridge. "In which," I read, "the whole circle of human learning is explained and the difficulties attending the acquisition of every art are removed in the most easy and familiar manner."

Published in the early 1800s, the leather spine was beginning to flake.

After mum's death I interviewed Dr. Hegarty about her conversation with mum. In an easy Irish lilt she remembered that "your mother was really feeling very low and she said 'I'm a bit of a nuisance, aren't I?' And I said, 'No, there are two things I think about you. You are very stoic and you're also very reasonable.' And she was delighted with that, but it was true. And her face kind of lit up." For all my complicated feelings about mum, I wear those words like a warm sweater.

The next day I called my father and, sure enough, mum had gone off to the hospital without a backward glance. I resolved to go that evening but in the meantime scrambled to divert myself with the final editing of an article chronicling certain of my doings in Buenos Aires, niggling over changes in syntax and wording that otherwise I'd have let go.

When I finally arrived at the Salvation Army Hospital, a nondescript red brick structure at the top of Church Street, I ran into my aunt Janet and Aubrey Russell, the long-time family solicitor. (Aubrey is a gentleman. Every year when he calls to remind me about my taxes, he refers to the payment as "meeting your obligation to Her Majesty.") The conversation was strange and not a little contrived. Aubrey suggested the family legend that we were blood relations to North American Indians was proved by my mother's carved features. Janet took Aubrey up on this point, insisting that it was a family myth. I tried to follow but soon grew impatient and excused myself to go upstairs.

What I saw when I entered her room threw me. Mum lay in bed looking—and there is no other word for it—cadaverous, her lower lip falling away at an odd angle in an upside-down sneer. For some reason the nursing staff had dressed her in an awful polyester nightie. The horrible tableau was completed by a cheap blue ribbon tied in a bow at her throat.

I sat down at the head of the bed and on autopilot told her I'd run into Janet and Aubrey in the waiting room. Mum looked straight ahead and said in a voice that seemed to have travelled a long distance over still water, "Dear, sweet Aubrey." These were the final words my mother spoke in my presence.

The blinds were drawn. I sat at the head of the bed regarding my mother, whose features did suddenly seem sculpted and ancient. I looked away, I can't be sure for how long. I can't remember what I was thinking, but when I looked back, mum was staring at me vulture-like, barely able to hold her eyes open. I reached for her and said, "Hi mummy," and she lifted her head up and closed her eyes. The effort to hold her head upright proved too much and her face fell away from me.

The room was painted a hideous pink. There was a plaque from the Rotary Club in loving memory of somebody or other, an ugly painting from the hot mush school of landscapes, and a generic poster of a cruise ship. All very "soothing."

I drifted out to the nursing station, where I discovered that Rita Temelkof had sent roses. At least they might provide relief from the room's relentless mediocrity. I was directed to a storage room containing an array of cut glass bowls and vases. As I scanned them, I was reassured by the idea that whatever other failures I might have in this life, selecting an appropriate vase or bowl on this occasion wouldn't be one of them.

I took the vase back in, having arranged the roses. Mum seemed to be dozing, so I left again, this time to call the office. I spoke to my editor. All the mistakes I had left to be "fixed" were still in the manuscript. I began to berate him. "This," I said, "is im*poss*ibly bad . . . inexcusable . . . *dizz*gusting."

"Jesus, what's your problem?" the voice on the other end of the phone inquired. "You sound like some sort of English biddy or something."

My mother had inhabited me and I'd been caught out.

I walked slowly back to the room, past a woman in thick glasses and a ratty plaid housecoat who was complaining about her "situation." She had a narrow ferret face and her eyes moved around looking for another soul from whom to elicit agreement. "I'm twice as sick as anyone else on this ward," she announced. Her goggle eyes stared at me as I passed. She was dying and that was my only comfort.

I sat with mum. Her breathing was laboured and rapid, and she was licking her lips constantly; a drop of saliva would form on her lips and periodically she'd spit it away. Until just that moment I could never have imagined my mother spitting. I became agitated sitting there, and found myself heading back to the lounge to call my dad. A family sat on the couch holding each other, watching *Wheel of Fortune*. I called to ask dad if mum would be alone through the evening, in a place I didn't think suited her. Dad sounded terribly tired. He said something vaguely reassuring and rang off.

I went back to her room. As I passed the nursing station, a voice called after me, "Your mum is just getting washed up and having her dressing changed. Ted's in there with her."

"Ted?" I thought.

I walked to the door. Behind it I could hear the sounds of a woman at the end of her life enduring the indignities of a rote procedure. I heard my mother moan in a way that indicated to me that she would be screaming blue murder if she could. I put my forehead against the door. For a moment I contemplated havoc.

Instead, I turned on my heel and walked down the hall. I stopped at the nursing station. I spoke quietly. "How many nurses work on the night shift?" I asked.

The woman had one of those indeterminately haggard female faces. Forty years of misery? Sixty? "Share your name," she said.

"Sorry?" I replied.

"Share your name with me, son."

Somewhere between my bowel and my spleen I heard a voice saying, "Share my name with you, you insect? I should think *not*." Luckily, this didn't find its way to my lips. Instead, I bowed in an oddly formal fashion—a carbon copy of my father in fact—and said, "Douglas Bell, ma'am. And I was wondering if you could tell me how many nurses might be on staff this evening should my mother need assistance during the night."

The number seemed grossly inadequate.

Just then events started to race ahead of me and I fled. Mumbling something to the nurse, I made a beeline for the elevator. In my mind was a tortured logic: I had to get home to call Jean and the kids, who'd gone to Ottawa for Thanksgiving. (I could just as easily have phoned them from the floor.) I practically fell into the lobby, where I found myself chatting to a glassed-in receptionist. I asked about the hours, when the place opened for visitors. Something in my manner must have tipped her off. She'd probably seen it a hundred, a thousand times before.

"You know, you can stay here longer if you like. Those hours listed don't apply to the immediate family."

"No, I have to go tend to my kids. They're away, you see. In Ottawa. I need to call my wife."

"There are phones there on that wall. You could call from here."

"No, no, it's okay, I . . ." I ran out through the sliding doors into a parking lot that backed onto Bloor Street.

I grabbed at the air for breath. Gazing through the darkness, I watched a man and woman with their arms linked hop cheerily down the stairs to the Plaza movie theatre. I wondered what was playing. Then I turned around and walked back inside, rode the elevator to the tenth floor, marched past the nursing station and into mum's room.

I'm told I owe the reader, at this stage, an explanation for my behaviour: coming and going, incapable of sitting still with my dying mother. The best I can do is to suggest I was in the grip of indecision regarding a situation over which I had no control. In the face of that, I played at my own private Godot.

They'd changed mum out of the hideous nightie into a purple hospital gown. It looked as though they'd washed her hair.

A water stain formed a halo around her head. Or was it sweat?

She was sleeping. Asleep, her expression was peaceful. She looked more alive than when she'd been awake.

The fluorescent lights in the room fought the night's encroaching gloom.

I sat with her a long time, sunk in her calm expression. Her breathing had slowed somewhat and her concentrated effort to expectorate had passed.

Ten o'clock came and went. I spoke in an even voice. "I'll be back first thing, mummy, I'll see you then."

I took a cab home. I lay in bed a long time unable to sleep. One thought kept tromping through my head. I needed a suit. I just thought I needed a suit. I decided in the midst of a long night that I would go first thing in the morning to Holt Renfrew and buy a suit. I knew exactly what kind of suit I wanted—conservative, navy blue, two pieces, three buttons, all seasons. A suitable suit. Every other thought that passed through my mind that night I found thoroughly disquieting, but not the idea of the suit.

I finally dropped off to sleep at five a.m. My last conscious thought was that I would need to buy a decent white hanky to go with the suit since I likely wouldn't be able to find mine.

My eyes popped open. "Have I got enough money for a suit?" I got on the phone to Jean in Ottawa, who told me that indeed I had enough for a suit. As regards anything practical, anything of consequence, I rely on Jean to give my life an imprimatur of reality. I knew the money was there, I just needed Jean to confirm that the money was *there*.

As an afterthought I mentioned that I didn't think mum was doing too well. Jean must have asked me a bunch of panicky questions, but I don't remember. I had to be at the hospital by ten-thirty when visiting hours began. And before that I needed to get to the men's department at Holt Renfrew.

It was just after nine-thirty when I walked through the doors, past the faux Beefeater and a noxious woman looking to squirt perfume at me. I went downstairs to the men's department, where I met a trim, compact fellow, a Mr.

Barlow. "Barlow is my grandmother's maiden name," I volunteered. He had a neatly trimmed moustache, polished loafers and razor-sharp creases in his trousers.

He pointed to several suits he thought fit the bill, then ceased his sales pitch almost instantly; he knew that I knew exactly what I wanted. He quickly produced a handsome shirt as white as the breaking surf on a sunny day, and a cheerfully patterned maroon tie. He gave me his card and heartily shook my hand as I made my way towards the hospital, four blocks along Bloor Street. I walked in the clear light, the Holt Renfrew bag swinging beside me.

In the hospital lobby I checked in again with the woman behind the glass. I was twenty minutes early for visiting hours. She told me not to fret—I could go right up. I got off the elevator and went round the corner away from my mother's room, dropping the shirt and tie off in the lounge. What was the point of showing them off without the suit?

As I made my way into my mother's room, I ran into dad coming the other way. He was weeping. I had never seen my father cry.

"I don't think she's going to survive this," he said, his head bowed forward into his hands, which were laid in a supplicant fashion along his cheeks.

I went into the room and sat in a chair a couple of feet from the end of the bed. My mother's features seemed stretched, as though her skin were being pulled up from the base of her neck. Her eyes were half open. There was something gnarled and overgrown about her lashes, almost as if they were tied together to prevent her from opening her eyes fully. I imitated my dad, sitting ramrod straight, shoulders square, legs at exactly the same angle as the legs of the chair.

Dad had followed me back in and stared absently at the window. He said, "I doubt she can even hear what we're saying."

There was a terrible noise from my mother's chest and her whole body seemed to groan. Yet she remained still.

Dad said something like, "Do you suppose that's it?"

I asked whether he thought I should go for a nurse.

"Yes," he said cautiously, "but they must do nothing heroic to save her. Your mother was very explicit about that."

Still, I felt as though I had to be at least purposeful in informing the nurses that my mother had died. Yes, that's it, I thought, she's died. That's what I'll tell them, that my mother has died, yes.

I came upon two nurses in the hallway. "Would you come quickly please? I think, I believe . . ." Yes, I remember thinking, that's right, because I'm not sure she's dead, how can I be? ". . . that my mother has just died."

I chased the nurses back down the hall and into the room. They looked to me as if they were going about their business with a certain urgency. Dad and I stood off to one side, watching as one nurse lowered the head of mum's bed and the other stared into her eyes and held her wrist. I looked past her through the blinds to the morning light beyond.

As I stared out through the slats at the green tinted windows of the office building across the street, something happened. It was like this: When you go to the optometrist to get your eyes checked, they sit you down in front of what appears to be a pair of binoculars. You look through the eyepiece and the doctor asks you to read the bottom line. Then they spin a variety of lenses in front of your eyes until they get the right one. You know the drill:

"Read the bottom line."

click

"Better?"

click

"Better?"

And eventually one lens clarifies your field of vision.

Standing there beside my dead mother as the nurses lowered the head of the bed sufficiently to lay her body flat, I heard it . . .

"click"

and the lens through which I saw my life unfurl before me in time's rolling scrolling chaos clicked and the world was . . . different. Not better, maybe worse, but palpably changed. I remember blinking a couple of times just to be sure.

And with that my father and I started a sort of relay grieving, each of us shuttling into the bathroom so as not to burden the other with our muffled sobs. Each time we came and went, the one would touch the other's shoulder.

You're it.

Then dad started to collect the things in the room. There was a book, of course, *A Gentleman Publisher's Commonplace Book* by John Murray, and a package of upscale British magazines. Reading *Country Life* one day, dead the next. As he did this, one of the nurses said, kindly I thought, "There's no need to rush out. Stay as long as you feel you need to."

Just then I felt very young. I replied in a small voice, "I'm going to stay with my father just at the moment, thank you."

Dad inhaled sharply through his nose and raised himself, shoulders squared and back ramrod straight. "Yes, yes," he said, affirming something. "Thank you. We'll be off now."

He turned to the door and pulled it towards him, and just as we crossed the threshold I heard myself say, "Bye bye mummy."

We walked down to the car and drove back to the apartment. I could see that dad needed to lay some weight on my shoulders—phone calls, arrangements, things that had to be done. First, though, we needed to find the missive from my mother laying out exactly how things were to go, how her death was to be marked. In his exhaustion dad forgot where he'd put it, so we called Aubrey Russell, who read it to me over the phone. I dutifully took it all down.

It was titled "Memorandum to my family and executors." As Aubrey read, I started to laugh at the turns of phrase, each of which reflected my mother's specific taste and unbending will. "I desire that my body be cremated in as simple and inexpensive a slab or box as can be obtained . . . a small early evening memorial service on the day of my death . . . the briefest standard Anglican burial service . . . the casket is not to be at the service."

Mum didn't want us to spend any more than necessary, not because she was parsimonious but because she thought funeral homes were rip-off artists and she was going to get hers back from beyond the grave. She even directed the proprietor to spread the ashes himself so that he might work for his pound of flesh. The brief and spare nature of the service she demanded reminded me of her behaviour during every funeral we had ever attended. Eulogies were always described by the same stock phrase: "He/she did go on some." Mother thought the business of rolling the casket up the aisle after the service was barbaric. And she'd always said she'd have none of it when the time came.

All this passed through my mind as Aubrey read. Then he informed me that mum had appointed me sole executor, her last crack at forcing me to tuck in my shirt. Dad had me call my half-sister, Patricia, and several others. For the most part people cried and thanked me profusely for calling. Patricia said something about having expected the news but that it still came as a shock. She soon turned up at the apartment with her latest beau, and we settled in for a drink before lunch.

Patricia asked my father something or other about the dispensation of mother's worldly goods. In a cool and gracious fashion he told her to direct her questions to me, as I would be handling things. "You're the sole executor?" she said, lacing her voice with dinner theatre incredulity.

My voice was toneless in response. "I'll have a clearer idea what's going on after I speak to Aubrey. You can give me a call after that."

During lunch I told the story of mother packing me off to eastern Europe with cartons and cartons of dried low-fat soup. Dad chuckled away.

The next day I accompanied dad to the funeral home to attend to the details regarding the disposal of mother's remains. We were ushered into a darkly panelled office and made to wait. I commented on the subdued, solicitous tone that everyone seemed to assume with "the bereaved" as regards "the beloved." Dad looked at me with the ever so slightly amused expression that indicates something really dry and funny is on the way. "Wait," he said. "You will not believe what you're about to hear."

Sure enough, moments later, the "arranging director" of the funeral home made his entrance. He had about him a comic gravitas. My dad and I had to sign a whole series of papers condemning mother's body to a fiery end followed by the spreading of her ashes on the grounds of Mount Pleasant Cemetery. The longer the man spoke in his sombre tones, the more he reminded me of the Disney version of Ichabod Crane. The same slightly stooped, goofy demeanour, the same bobbing Adam's apple.

There were two rich highlights in all this. The first came when dad and I had to descend into the bowels of the building to select, as per my mother's instructions, the least expensive box. The arranging director waved his hand over every casket in the place, describing in rich detail the features of each. Something playing around one corner of my dad's mouth kept me from interrupting. Finally the director came to a relatively unadorned, plain brown casket. "This," he said, "is our lowest-priced model." Then dad, barely gesturing into one corner of the room, asked about that one there. Ichabod turned sharply, as though he'd been stung by a bee from behind. Sure enough, invisible to all but the sharpest eye was what looked to be a particleboard box.

"My wife's instructions were explicit." Dad looked over at me, his eyes mad with pleasure. "You would agree?"

"Sure, yes. I mean, yes, absolutely."

Ichabod led us out without a word, back upstairs to the office. "Now," he said, having placed himself back behind his desk and laid his hands flat on the blotter, "we'll need to have someone identify Mrs. Bell."

I looked over at my father. His expression shadowed my thought. "Why would we need to do that?"

It turns out there is a government regulation. I jumped up before he'd finished his citation. "Let's get on with it, shall we?"

I followed his every solemn step . . . down . . . each . . . and . . . every . . . stair. Then the door was opened and there was my mother's body. Her lips gave off a glossy white sheen as though they'd been smeared with Vaseline. I heard Ichabod's voice saying something sombre and understanding.

In that moment you might imagine that time would stand still, but it did not. In fact, it suddenly accelerated. My course was clear. I turned back instantly and pushed my shoulder into his chest. Having made a hole for myself, I fled back up the stairs. "Yes," I said without turning back, "that's her."

By the time the service rolled around on Monday evening, things had taken a somewhat zigzag course. We had hoped to enlist John Erb, the former minister at Grace Church on the Hill. Mum had arranged flowers at that church at John Erb's request, and Erb had presided over my daughter Charlotte's baptism. But he was unavailable, so we ended up with an earnest young fellow with a suitable pedigree (a degree from Trinity College), who retained the impression—despite my best efforts at disabusing him—that he was there to lead us through our grief. At one point in the course of a service that otherwise would have fit the bill ("the briefest standard Anglican burial service") our man decided to talk about how it is we come to reconcile ourselves to death in the course of a Christian life. At least I think that's what he talked about. After a couple of minutes all I could feel was heat rising like steam out of a New York City sewer on an August day. He went on and on and on, and I could barely look around the room for fear I'd start to giggle. I felt my mother's impatience there in the room: "He *is* going on some."

At least the prayers were comforting. "I believe in God the Father Almighty, Maker of heaven and earth: And in Jesus Christ his only Son our Lord, Who was conceived by the Holy Ghost, Born of the Virgin Mary, Suffered under Pontious Pilate, Was crucified, dead, and buried, He descended into hell; The third day he rose again from the dead, He ascended into heaven, And sitteth at the right hand of God the Father Almighty; From thence he shall come to judge the quick and the dead. I believe in the Holy Ghost; The holy Catholic Church; The Communion of Saints; the Forgiveness of sins; The Resurrection of the body; And the Life everlasting. Amen"

That bit about the forgiveness of sins cut both ways. Mum saved me and I couldn't save her. If you ask me, I believe in the forgiveness of sins. I hope mum did too.

In the end, everyone thought the service was fine. The suit went over well and I managed to keep my shirt-tail tucked in. Afterwards we sat about and told lighthearted stories, and ate cucumber and salmon sandwiches, my mother's death just one more obstacle around which the tepid conversation had to wend its way.

On the way home Charlotte, who was six, piped up from the back. "You never told me that granny, you know . . . died." Earlier in the day, just after Jean, Charlotte and Anne returned from Ottawa, I had taken Charlotte aside and trotted out the thin gruel about death that I'd been fed at her age. "Granny has gone up into heaven. She's got a beautiful garden to tend there and she's very happy . . ." But this tissue of fabrications was soon shredded, and Charlotte was clearly miffed at having been shunted onto a spur away from truth's main line.

Several months later—March 19, 1999, to be exact—my elder daughter arranged some objects she'd found around the house on the dining-room table, the centrepiece of which was a framed portrait of my mother. "It's for Granny," Charlotte said. "She'd like it." I made a list of the contents in my notebook under the heading "The Oddest Thing":

> Charlotte made a shrine for my mother. A silver tray, tulip stalks and tulip petals neatly separated, a wooden elephant taken from a child's puzzle, five tea cups and saucers, a pair of tiny red Barbie sunglasses, a glass candlestick, various shells, a starfish and several raisin-oatmeal cookies, surrounding a framed reproduction of my mother's portrait. Around one of the tulip stalks was one of my wife's silver rings. Charlotte saw me writing in my notebook and asked to sign her name on the page on which I recorded these details.

AFTERMATH

> It was drizzling and mysterious at the beginning of our journey. I could see that it was all going to be one big saga of the mist. "Whooee!" yelled Dean. "Here we go!" And he hunched over the wheel and gunned her; he was back in his element, everybody could see that. We were all delighted, we all realized we were leaving confusion and nonsense behind and performing our one and noble function of the time, move.
>
> —JACK KEROUAC, *On the Road*

SO WHAT DO YOU DO WHEN the thing you weren't prepared for changes everything in your life and yet you spend your time imagining you're handling it just fine, thank you very much? First you read and then you travel, thinking that these activities will give you some control. Then, in the midst of that, other things happen that undo your tightly woven control. And that always fucks you up. In his novel *Scar Tissue*, Michael Ignatieff gets this tension exactly right:

> What happens can never be anticipated. What happens escapes anything you can ever say about it. What happens cannot be redeemed. It can never be anything than what it is. We tell stories as if to refuse this truth, as if to say we make our fate, rather than simply endure it. But in truth we make nothing. We live and we cannot shape life. It is much too great for us, too great for any words.

What I read

Before and after my mother died, I read obsessively about three things: illness, mortality and memory. The books seemed to turn in various degrees on any or all of these three subjects.

The best discussion I've ever read on what it's actually like to be mortally ill is *Intoxicated by My Illness*, a memoir of Anatole Broyard's cancer. In it he describes how to get on with your illness. He describes how to rise above it and be better than it is. He writes in a conversational manner, but what a conversation — funny, unlikely and canny. And he wrote these words, not from the safe quarters of recovery, but staring mortality in the face. How about this on what an illness amounts to: "To be ill is an odd mixture of pathos and bathos, comedy and terror, with intervals of surprise. To treat it too respectfully is to fall into the familiar florid traps of the romantic agony." And then: "illness is not all tragedy, much of it is funny."

There were other good books on the subject: Ignatieff's *Scar Tissue* (a memoir barely disguised as a novel); *Death Be Not Proud* by John Gunther; *A Leg to Stand On* by Oliver Sacks; *Patient* by Ben Watt; *The Diving Bell and the Butterfly* by Jean-Dominique Bauby. Each of them revealed to me a clue.

Ignatieff got his mother's death from Alzheimer's spot on. I read this passage with my feet soaking in the cool ultra-blue waters of Mono Lake just outside Banff, Alberta, when my own mother had only two months to live:

> If you believe that she knew we were there, if you believe—I cannot be sure—that she understood what her sons needed at that instant, her eyes which had been shut and which by being closed made her seem completely out of reach suddenly opened. Blue grey eyes with a hint of yellow in the iris, eyes now beyond sight, staring up into the ceiling above her son's heads, upward ever upwards, fixed like an exhausted swimmer on the shore.

The Diving Bell and the Butterfly falls into the you-think-you've-got-it-bad school of medical memoir. Bauby had a stroke that reduced his capacity for intentional movement to blinking his left eye, yet he manged to write an intelligent and self-effacing book about it. Oliver Sacks and Ben Watt produced, from wildly different perspectives, what are essentially illness *policiers*: books that go deep inside their mangled flesh. Sacks, best known for his books *Awakenings* and *The Man Who Mistook His Wife for a Hat*, writes about breaking his leg in a hiking accident and then losing for a time the capacity in any way to control his ruined pin. "This is what I had felt . . . the sense, the foreboding, that the muscle was dead. It was, above all, its silence which conveyed this impression, a silence utter and absolute, the silence of death." Ben Watt, whose day job is as one-half of the pop duo Everything But The Girl, writes a memoir of a rare disease that eats away at his small intestine. This book introduced me to a sort of inadvertent twin, in that his misery too centres on his gut: "For the next 24 hours, whenever I felt nauseous, a nurse would aspirate the tube, drawing the bile out with a large plastic syringe. I would watch it run down the tube from my nose. Sometimes it would be pale and yellow, like finger bowl water. Other times it would come up thick and green and full of sediment, like pond algae or mint sauce." I could, as they say, relate.

Death Be Not Proud is a book so charged and moving that it is almost unbearable to read. Written by his father, it is the story of Johnny Gunther, a brilliant teenager who succumbs to a brain tumour over the course of a year or so. The book is broken into two parts: John Gunther's account of his son's illness and death, followed by excerpts from his son's letters and diaries. The diaries are especially poignant in that they reveal a young mind that grasped fundamental moral truths in the face of mortality. He expresses them in a clear, unaffected prose from which no writer could fail to learn. "Happiness," the doomed teen writes, "depends on moderation—not too much ambition—humility—don't give a damnness."

Currently, the world's heavyweight champion in the death and dying division is *Tuesdays with Morrie* by Mitch Albom. If you haven't at least heard of it, you've likely been living among the Taliban for the last three years. Morrie Schwartz is an academic who finds himself dying of ALS, or Lou Gehrig's disease, and subsequently becomes something of a national celebrity thanks to a series of reflective interviews with Ted Koppel as his condition deteriorates. Throughout the terminus course of his illness Morrie meets with a former student, Mitch Albom, to discuss the unresolved questions of the age.

Morrie is not the problem here. He comes off as a decent fellow struggling with the questions that need to be asked in the face of his imminent death. The problem is Albom, who seeks to comfort his readers in the face of their most profound imperfection: that they are going to die. It's a conjuring trick. What Morrie summed up in fourteen weeks, Albom feeds back to us in bite-sized chunks, as Morrie's gift to the world. Death renders him perfect. I suspect that deep in their hearts those who read this book know it's a cheat, that ambiguity is the genuine condition of death and fate. No matter how pleasantly packaged, death, in the end, is a reign of terror that we must confront and embrace, more like Morrie, less like Mitch.

The things that drive you to madness

Within a few weeks of mum's finale I was confronted by two more deaths. And whereas I now imagined I had the experience to know how to behave, the discrete nature of death rendered me confused and miserable.

The first was a colleague from my days at the business magazine. He attended my wedding. We played hockey together once a week for several years. He was up from absolutely nothing. His father had been a cook in the Canadian military. He'd just turned thirty-nine, and his heart stopped in the middle of the night. For weeks thereafter his kids stuck their noses into his closet to smell his essence in the folds of his pants and shirts and coats. The funeral was just plain sad, grey and sad. The efforts at hearty reminiscence quickly gave way after the service to drunkenness at a local bar.

Several weeks after that a close friend's mother died after falling down the stairs. An American of torrentially high spirits, she was known to all as Joey. There was a service up in Ottawa at the same small Anglican church in which Jean and I had been married. At the service various people got up and spoke about Joey. There were funny stories, touching stories, hardly any maudlin stories. Mum, I thought, if only she'd had the patience, might have enjoyed it. Afterwards there was a mad party at the Château Laurier. Joey's American cousins were riotous good fun.

Just before the service, my friend approached me. I reached for something stirring to say. After all, I was an old hand. "Batten down the hatches, Ken," was all I could come up with.

Where you wander

About a year after my mother died, I decided to take a tour of the American cities I'd passed through before and during my hospitalization for pancreatitis in 1990, two weeks on the road reconstructing a trip that almost killed me. I thought this time away might afford me some distance from my mourning, distance that might provide me with perspective. It seemed like I'd spent the whole year trying to find a lost love. At the same time, I wondered whether this wasn't inherently fruitless, since you can't find love by conscious effort. It has to find you.

My mother, fierce and scary though she could be, gave absolutely everything she had in an effort to save me when I got hit by that truck. She would have put herself in my place. She'd have died for me. That, I sense, is love. But because I'm a man and she was my mother, I spent the next twenty-odd years trying to put distance between us so I could prove myself to myself. In doing this I lost my faith in her love and sought instead *accomplishments*– jobs, wife, children, prestige—all the while checking over my shoulder, trying to catch her eye. "See what I did. How about that?"

Then she was dying of cancer, and then she was dead. And I started to wonder what was *that* all about? I mean, she's dead and there's nobody to please now but myself. There's the love I feel for my wife and children, but the fact is, even *they* were partly about pleasing my mother and to some extent protecting me from illness and my own chaotic behaviour. For the moment it felt like a kind of double jeopardy: those things that were there for the purpose of proving myself worthy of my mother's love are disqualified from being put to this new purpose—defining myself as somehow apart, separate, distinct. An embarrassing, pitiful admission for a forty-year-old man but vividly accurate nonetheless.

As my mother receded from this world, it was like a door opened onto another world that might have been or could still be if only I were somebody else. But, according to the rules, all I was supposed to do was stand in the doorway and look. Okay, so I did a little more than look. (And that's all I'm going to say about that. In *The Bend for Home*, his memoir of growing up Irish, Dermot Healy writes, "Can I lie here and sidestep some memory I'd rather not entertain and then let fiction take care of it elsewhere, because that is sometimes what fiction does? It becomes the receptacle for those truths we would rather not allow into our tales of the self.")

I was so startled and terrified by my behaviour that all I had left was this book. So I took a trip, ostensibly to investigate the nature of love by remembering what it's like to pray for my life to be spared. I was seeking an ill-defined epiphany, always a lousy idea. And then the way things are with me, it all turned into a random jumble.

I arrived in Vancouver and went immediately to visit Mike Guy. He was living in Gibsons Landing, a relatively isolated community on the north shore of Howe Sound, accessible only by a forty-minute ferry ride. Mike and I share a common fault: we like to fall in love. After getting his three sons to bed, we spent the night drinking Scotch and discussing it—love, that is. We came to no conclusions.

The next day I retraced my steps to the UBC campus, through the Museum of Anthropology and down to Wreck Beach. I stood looking at the ridiculous view and feeling not much besides the increasing chill as the sun dropped quickly away on a late fall afternoon.

At noon the next day I lunched with a famous author. He drove me from my hotel to the Stanley Park teahouse in his gleaming new Audi sports coupe. By any standard he qualifies as rich and famous, a sage for a generation, and though I tried to put it all to the side of my mind, I couldn't really. Over lunch I talked too much about myself, then tried to salvage things by seeking his advice and guidance regarding . . . me.

"You'd be extremely dangerous inside a corporation," he said. "You could go random at any time."

I was meant to be off to Seattle the next day, but I was delayed when I took up my twin cousin Geoff's offer for lunch, which then turned into golf, which in turn transformed into a night on the town. Geoff was in the middle of a miserable divorce that involved not only the active alienation of his ex-wife but the possibility of his children drifting away as well. She wanted her fair share not just of Geoff's assets and income derived from his work as a financier, but of his considerable family fortune too.

Returning to his newly minted bachelor-parent pad, I reminded him that his wife had pitched him out the same weekend my mother died. Geoff had been in the midst of a golfing holiday, and he said he remembered the trip well. His eyes glazed over as he reported that on the return leg of the journey, on his way to finding that the locks had been changed, he had travelled first class on British Airways. "You can stretch out and go to sleep, for Chrissakes. And with the points it was actually cheaper than if I'd flown business class.

"That," he went on almost dreamily, "was a great trip."

I felt for him then. Despite his moneyed bravado, I could see that the whole thing had left him with a dead spot inside. It hardly mattered that Geoff wasn't giving voice to his pain. He was in that moment the archetypal male stoic. And there was for me—a rushing river of barely contained emotion—a lesson in that.

I arrived in Seattle in the midst of the sort of soggy, cloudy, closed-in conditions that reinforce the city's stereotype. I retraced my steps to the bed and breakfast above Pyke's market and walked out First Avenue through Pioneer Square to the Kingdome. Just as I arrived, a Seahawks game was letting out, and I repeated the walk back into town in almost exactly the same circumstances as nine years earlier. As I walked, I felt a rising anxiety that I associated with my attack.

Then it was on to Newport by way of Portland, the city from which Jean and I had started our flight from hell. Portland was terrific. Tons of gorgeous trees line the downtown streets, and they were particularly beautiful thanks to the fall colours. While there, I had dinner with a friend, Jonathan Brinckman, a Pulitzer Prize–nominated environmental reporter for *The Oregonian*. Jonathan also has a degenerative disease, and I could see that his condition was deteriorating. He was slurring his words a titch and was a little unstable on his feet. But there's not an ounce of self-pity about him. He talked about how he's trying to rethink his life to make the best use of his time. It was obvious what he was talking about. Jonathan possesses the sort of grace in the face of physical diminution that I would have wanted for myself if I hadn't been so panicked by it all.

The next morning I was on my way to Newport, where I'd been hospitalized. In the absence of pain, the ride down on the bus was amazing. We drove through the rich mossy greens of the coastal forest and then along the wild, craggy coast. The surf was really up, the wash extending five hundred yards or so out into the Pacific. Just as we pulled into Newport, I saw one of those blue hospital signs by the highway and jerked up in my seat.

I was dropped at a little shack by the interstate, just a hundred yards from the low-slung hospital building. I followed my nose a mile and a half or so back to the Embarcadero, where my wife had stayed. I passed the restaurant, Vic's Waterfront Café, where I felt the first stirrings of the awful pain. I walked on to the motel beside the port's forest of ship masts and tangle of fishing paraphernalia. I settled in, rented a bike and headed back up to the hospital. There I applied for my records and revisited the floor on which I'd stayed. I remembered the view out over the plain seaside motels across the coastal highway from the hospital. Beyond that, I seemed to be more or less sleepwalking.

As I had to wait an hour and a half for my records, I decided to get some lunch at the Newport restaurant and lounge across the way. It was a typical roadside joint with lots of wood panelling, and displayed prominently on one wall was a life-size inflatable shark with a football jammed into its snout. And then the random nature of things (or at least the random nature of what I find interesting) took hold. As I sat down I was considering the news that Dr. Beemer was now a coroner. As I contemplated the possibility of going to visit him, a couple settled into the booth behind me. I was in a far corner of the restaurant and they may have failed to notice me. They obviously thought themselves beyond anyone's earshot. I found myself taking notes of the conversation.

The couple had just returned from giving evidence at a hearing of a local grand jury into whether or not to indict the woman's ex-husband or lover, and they had come to the restaurant for lunch and a few drinks to relax. They both ordered doubles. The first part of the conversation that entered my consciousness was the boyfriend saying, "I never choked her. I grabbed her by the throat to restrain her when she attacked me. I did slap her with an open palm after she stabbed me in the stomach. I was sound asleep when she stabbed me in the stomach."

The woman responded with soap-opera bitchiness, "Do you mind if I give you some advice . . . take it or leave it." She bit those words off so harshly that I couldn't concentrate on the advice itself.

The conversation turned back to the proceedings at the grand jury: assessments of the prosecutors, the other witnesses and the central character in all this drama, her ex. The issue seemed to be whether the indictments returned by the grand jury would issue in a sentence long enough to keep him out of her hair.

Then their talk took a strange, fascinating, chilling turn. The woman: "You're not going to believe it when you hear the tapes. You're going to think I'm crazy playing up to him the way I did. It's what I had to say to pacify him. I can't believe I'm this stupid. He's never going to stop unless I kill him. I just can't do that."

The boyfriend's tone turned angry. "You've got to stop showing remorse. Stop feeling sorry for yourself or him. Man, I'd like to take a shot at him."

Her tone became coquettish and challenging. "I'd love for you to fight him. Though he's strong. He's tall and skinny, but he's strong. I'm strong, but when he put me down he put me down hard. I'm not sure you could handle him."

Jesus, I thought, she's baiting him.

"I can handle him," he growled.

"I hope so, because he's telling people on the inside that he's sorry. That he wants me back. And there are people that are enabling him in that."

Nice: you better kill the guy or I might go back to him.

Moments later they got up from their booth to play pinball. I slouched down as they passed, then rose and made a beeline for the door. The boyfriend eyed me as I passed.

I peeled out of there on my bike and back to the hospital, where I picked up my medical records. But I couldn't get the couple's conversation out of my mind. I clambered back on the bike and, as I headed back to the motel, stopped at the hospital heliport, a square blacktop mound with landing lights and a windsock. Embedded at the western foot of the mound was a bronze plaque. It read simply:

Pacific Communities Hospital Heliport.
Promoted by the fishermen's wives of Newport

in memory of
Lawrence Andrew Jincks
William Norman Hallowel
Jim Harold McDow
Lost from the fishing vessel *Miss Corrine*
On March 5, 1979
And all other fishermen lost at sea.

I started to cry. I read it again and felt weightless, floating in no particular direction. And as I floated, some guy who beat his lover was going to get killed and I was angry with some doctors and these fishermen died. And I thought of the wives of those fishermen. How horrible. And I thought of my mother and how, when she died, a window opened on that other world and I could reach for it but I couldn't touch it, because the world I was in included a wife and two girls and a dog and a mortgage. And I live in that world because I am my mother's son.

And then I thought about the murderous woman and her dupe. Had they realized I'd been listening?

I rushed back to the motel, where I stayed up most of the night waiting to catch the five a.m. bus back to Portland. At the sound of the alarm I gathered my stuff up and headed for the lobby to meet my taxi. Of course, as it turned out, the motel had forgotten to change the clocks back from daylight savings to standard time, so I had an hour to kill. I ended up chatting with the night porter, who told me of his grand plan to retrofit a defunct luxury liner as a combination commercial fishing boat and floating processor. He planned to take the whole ball of wax to the South Pacific to fish for tuna and live out the rest of his days on an island in Micronesia. He told me this story while changing the letters on the motel bulletin board to announce that the local chapter of Toastmasters would be meeting that morning at ten.

Eventually the cab arrived and I was on my way. The bus station in Newport is little more than a fake-wood-panelled shack alongside the highway. It was pouring with rain, and as I waited for my bus a variety of my fellow passengers stumbled onto the scene. Two of the four had a tattooed teardrop etched in the skin at the corner of one eye.

In one corner of the shack stood a bookstand featuring twenty or so titles, which I browsed till the bus arrived. All the books were published by Focus on the Family, a Christian group dedicated to promoting family life lived along biblical lines. My favourite title was *Sportin' a 'Tude: What Your Attitude Says When You're Not Looking* by Patsy Clairmont. The cover featured sixty-something Patsy decked out in a fire-engine red leather suit, striking a series of poses that I think were meant to illustrate the various 'tudes to which she took exception in the book.

Soon the bus turned up and we piled on to avoid the rain. Three blocks later we stopped in front of The Apple Peel diner, where everybody piled off for breakfast before starting off again an hour later. I felt compelled to ask why the bus would stop three blocks from the bus station when the schedule stated explicitly that it left Newport at five a.m. "Yeah," replied the bus driver, "weird, isn't it? But nobody around here seems to mind."

From Portland I flew to Chicago on the same flight I'd ruined for the other first-class passengers nine years before. This time I flew coach. From the airport I headed straight for the Resurrection Hospital. Same deal as Newport: the identical view from the hospital room, this time over flat and uninspired suburban Chicago. In the front lobby stood a painted statue of Jesus Christ complete with carved-out stigmata on the palms of his hands. I took notes of the statue's various features. Later I wished I'd turned to a couple of the volunteers standing nearby and pointed out that those wounds would probably require stitches.

Again I felt insubstantial. Rather than hang around the hospital I took off downtown and wandered among the towers and great doings of Chicago, hoping perhaps that the gravitas of the place might infuse me with a sense of purpose. I attended a talk by the travel writer Jan Morris in which she reprised a number of articles she'd written about cities throughout the world. Among these was a piece in which she claimed that living in Toronto was tantamount to winning second prize in the lottery of life.

That night, wandering around the lobby of the hotel trying to find a spot from which to watch the upcoming heavyweight championship fight, I ran into Frank Lazzaro, a roly-poly wholesale razor salesman. We decided to split the cab fare to a bar where the fight was showing. This in turn bought me a ringside seat to his life story.

Several years earlier, a benign tumour was discovered buried deep in the brain behind his eye. It was affecting his eyesight and because of its position could be treated only with radiation. He told this story in a broad Bronx accent and at first I found myself paying far more attention to the cadence and intonation of his speech than to the content. "So I go to dis doctor, high-flyin' reputation 'an all, and, like, he looks at me and says you're not one of dese Noo Yawkas dat needs five opinions, and I'm tinkin' I gotta tooma heeya and dis guy's givin' me attittoode." Well, it was certainly better than listening to the ins and outs of the razor business.

There was a moment in the conversation where I thought, here's where I can tell him of all my sicknesses and deaths, the common language of our experiences. Instead, while Lennox Lewis beat the tar out of Evander Holyfield on the surrounding screens, I let him go on about how after all his treatments he'd been brought back to the clinic at Harvard where he'd received his radiation treatment. One of his doctors wanted him to give a pep talk to a thirty-year-old, recently married cardiologist with exactly the same condition as Frank. "He was kinda down on himself, so I says to him, I says, You got too much at stake to give up. I mean, if you give up, you're probably giving some guy you don't even know a death sentence. And he saw what I was sayin' and he went ahead and got the radiation. And I feel like that's what I gave back."

And there I was in a bar in Chicago with a stranger, wondering whether I'd given anything back.

The next morning I woke up hung over and called my wife. I told her I was tired of travelling, missed the kids and wanted to come home.

That evening I stood on the steps of my house, luggage strewn about, hugging Anne. She leaned into me, her head turned to one side, nuzzling against my stomach. I bent from the waist and reached around her middle, pulling her into the air upside down. She squealed and I watched as her feet dangled in the air. And I sensed just then the wisdom trotted out to me by a friend whose life was . . . let's just say very complicated. "There's no secret to it, you know," she said.

"Yep," I thought. "Just my sweet little monkey's feet wagging back and forth, back and forth and my head bobbing to avoid a kick in the head, back and forth, back and forth."

My mind

The two events that twirled together to fire my memory and imagination—my accident and my mother's death—are like that, low-hanging chandeliers swinging back and forth along life's corridor. They light my way, but I need to duck constantly to avoid being cracked in the head.

As she died, my mother couldn't tell me about her pain and fear. She didn't want to; one simply didn't speak of it. As a consequence I never had the chance to balance the scales. She had comforted me at the moment of my greatest peril, but I was left with silence. It's hard to fault her. My mother didn't want to render me helpless, which I was when it came to her dying.

There are birds that feed along the shore near the apartment where I lived for a while on the California coast just south of Los Angeles. I watched them every morning spinning and whirling through the crashing surf. It always reminded me of something, though of what, I wasn't sure.

Later I came across a poem by Elizabeth Bishop, called "Sandpiper." It reads in part:

The roaring alongside he takes for granted,
and that every so often the world is bound to shake.
He runs, he runs to the south, finical, awkward,
in a state of controlled panic, a student of Blake . . .
looking for something, something, something.

Poor bird, he is obsessed!
The millions of grains are black, white, tan, and gray,
mixed with quartz grains, rose and amethyst.

That's me mimicking the ineluctable nature of the sandpiper, running harum-scarum into the feeding ground left by the receding wash, then running out again just ahead of the surging surf. In liminal moments we walk in among our grainy memories, like comical birds staring between our feet as life recedes, then skip out of the way as she crashes again, yet again, onto our shore.

My life

And what if you travel, read and seek some refuge in the certainties of wife and children, and muddle through everything else, and your mind's still a great heaving mess? That's easy. You go nuts. You fall deeply deeply in love with someone else. You indulge yourself in every misery your mind can conjure. You stop reading the newspaper. You look stricken and everyone feels bad for you—everyone, that is, except the people closest to you, your wife and kids, who think you're a jerk. Your mind wanders to the point that one spring evening, after working out for ninety minutes in an effort to relieve the constant cacophony between your ears, you mistakenly walk into the women's change room at a downtown Toronto health club and stand fiddling with the weigh scale. "I'm fat, oh Christ, I have to lose some more weight," you mumble, oblivious to the women who walk by staring daggers at you. Finally a voice reaches through the cotton in your brain—"Hey! . . . Hey! . . . What the fuck are you doing?" and you rush out, your face burning, and run down to the front desk to turn yourself in, imagining being hauled off in handcuffs.

And you want to admit everything: "My mum died and I loved her so much because she took care of me when I was sick and for a time it was as though I had lost my capacity to love at all. And then I fell in love with another woman. Oh god, oh god, oh god, I'm terribly terribly sorry. I must learn to love people for who they are and not for how they make me feel. I know that now. It took me forty years, but I figured it out. And no one's going to rescue me from myself. I must be responsible for my own happiness, for my actions. I need to believe it, sure, but somehow I have to live that way, too."

And the woman at the desk looks a little puzzled at what you're saying. In fact, you're not entirely certain yourself what you've just said.

"That's all right," she says, "no one seems to have complained."

Later still, I wrote this letter to a friend, betraying Dermot Healy's dictum: "It's August, worse yet it's the end of August. The air has that too ripe quality, sodden and thick with garbage smell. It's the kind of weather that merges all too easily with the mess I've made of my mind. For months now I've tortured my family and myself. My modus operandi is common to the point of banality. Two years ago mum died, at which point I started writing a book about that event and other matters pertaining to me: a terrible accident I suffered as a teenager, wretched debilitating illnesses that plagued me thereafter. Then in the midst of writing I had an affair. I fell in love with an astonishingly beautiful woman. I spent two weeks with her in a faraway city, ostensibly writing my book, and she told me stories about her Jewish family. Her grandfather was a tailor. Her mother was a venerated professional who'd died suddenly some years previous. I hung on her every word. All we talked about was love and death.

Thereafter exaltation swiftly turned to torment. I became confused. My life as I understood it up to then seemed pallid and undernourished. The possibility of another life beckoned; brighter, more vibrant, livelier. But I felt as though I was a long way down the chain of being, looking up. I had to choose. I failed to choose. As I failed I became mired in indecision, fretful and relentlessly unhappy. I became a source of pain and anguish for my wife and my children. My four-year-old kept asking why I shook so much. My eight-year-old took to making a beeping noise every time I came anywhere near her, as though I was a dump truck full of misery backing blindly into every room. My wife's anger and anxiety knew no limits. Lately I've had what's commonly referred to as a nervous breakdown. As a kid I heard my mother use this expression whenever things got ahead of her. It was an expression of panic, as in 'If you don't be quiet I'll have a nervous breakdown' or 'If I don't find my glasses this instant I'll have a nervous breakdown.'

My nervous breakdown was nothing like what I imagined from my mother's description, which I thought had something to do with chewing your nails and biting your lip a lot. I spent three days alternating between the floor of my shower and my bed. I screamed in the shower and moaned on the bed. At one stage I went into convulsions and my head hit the wall behind me like a jackhammer. I ended up on Valium. It came in the form of tiny blue pills slipped under the tongue like some suicide pill taken by downed spy plane pilots during the Cold War. As the pill dissolved, everything seemed to flatten out. And it was as though I didn't really care or half forgot what it was I was supposed to be worrying about. Later my psychiatrist suggested that overcoming my anxiety and confusion were rooted in my need to separate. Whether this was from my mother or my lover or my wife didn't really matter. I needed distance and perspective in order to go on. And though it seems ridiculous and melodramatic to me now, the fact is I did spend an afternoon riding the subway imagining I couldn't spend one more day feeling the way I did. So I decided not to. I decided not to feel suicidal, which points to the fact that I probably wasn't suicidal in the first place, just confused . . . which is the way I am . . . confused or lazy or if I'm feeling cocky I imagine that in fact I enjoy courting ambiguity, which is bullshit. But at least it's my bullshit."

And in the midst of all this we had scheduled a trip to Ireland as a family. And somehow we took it. Looking back, I can say that those nine days we spent together were really the only moments I've felt even remotely content in the two years since my mother died. Then of course there's this book—and as my mother used to say, the thing of it is, I'm beginning to wonder whether I'm writing the book or the book is writing me.

On a map of Ireland you'd identify our destination as the north shore of Clew Bay. Ecologists call it the Clew Bay Complex. According to an ecological description from which I draw this reference, it "encompasses a large area of open marine water and many islands along the Southwest coast of Mayo from Mulrany to Murrisk and supports a great diversity of both coastal and terrestrial habitats. The site is of international importance as an example of a drumlin landscape which formed during the last glacial period, when sediments were laid down and smoothed over by advancing ice—the sea has subsequently inundated this area, creating a multitude of islands in Clew Bay." All of which is true, but it doesn't quite get at the thing about the place that's true for me, which is that it is charismatic and odd and charming.

The place fires my imagination in two ways. First, it is stunningly beautiful. Anyone who crosses your line of sight is set against the backdrop of the sea, the ever-changing North Atlantic sky and the surrounding rock-strewn mountains—including Croagh Patrick, the holiest mountain in Christendom (okay, Irish Christendom)—and is improved by it. And anyone who speaks other than me, my family and the odd German visitor is issuing a natural poetry so touching and wry that it will, if you're not paying attention, cause you to weep. Say you happen to mention what a glorious day it is. Comes the reply: "Sure 'tis grand today, but it'll turn and we'll not see the sun for a month, that's for sure."

Among the variety of terrains on which I stood to observe all this, I loved the strand the best. The strand is a vast area of sandy tidal flats that's available for walking or running during several hours each day. Then slowly, slowly, relentlessly, the tide rolls in and fills the space between the furrows of sand until there is nothing left but a shoreline and ocean water. And for a second you wonder how it could ever go out again. So much water. And then it does, and since you can't watch the tides come and go in real time, you end up asking the same question again, only in reverse. How will the water ever fill that empty space again? And because I know it will, I go out to the strand and run.

Running on this vast expanse has an extraordinary aesthetic appeal. At sunset on a hazy day the mountains all around the bay turn a navy blue. And against the fading light of the pale pinky sky they resemble vast shadows cast up from the sea. The sandy expanse is bounded by tidal channels and pools that reflect that light. One evening as I ran, this light filled me with an overwhelming sense that its reflection bore my childhood. There was nothing specific that this feeling engendered, no particular memory, and yet in all its vagueness the feeling had two distinct and separate compartments. As I moved across the sand and watched that light dance in and out of the passing pools of water, I felt insubstantial against the vastness of the ocean swaying beyond the strand. That was the first compartment. And then as I continued, I entered the second compartment of feeling and was confronted—it was a much bigger compartment—by the harsh consequences of my behaviour. If I left, my wife would never forgive me. Understandably, she would turn my children against the woman I'd fallen in love with and by extension against me. This was the truth, and for all my efforts at explaining it to myself in an amber light, the truth would out and I would feel myself lesser for it. But—what was worse—if I did nothing, I felt somehow that I would in the end lose out not only to myself but also to some standard of beauty and sexuality that I hadn't the fortitude to pursue. Perhaps I was going the safe route, the route that made it appear as though I was looking out for my children, and in fact it was all just fear. And yet I kept running and I kept not deciding, every evening. Nothing changed and anything could distract me.

On the last day of our holiday, towards the end of my last run, I see something on the sand, formations that resemble small plates of spaghetti and are known as wormcasts. They dot the strand every three or four feet. They are formed when the worms living in the ground swirl to the surface. The remnant is literally cast in sand. At any rate, as I run, I see one being formed and it stops me in my tracks as I watch the swirling pattern emerge. And when I run on, I am suddenly thinking of everything: of lovers left behind, a wife spurned, children unattended and work left undone. And this, I now sense, is really what we leave in our wake as we go. Remnants. The rest—the triumphant self-justifications, this or that grand edifice of logic, the arguments to and fro and for and against—is what we want to be remembered for. But it's what we don't manage, what we leave to chance, what we say when we aren't paying attention—these are the things that define us and frame us.

These lines from "Tintern Abbey" get at this sensibility exactly:

> I bounded o'er the mountains, by the sides
> Of the deep rivers, and the lonely streams,
> Wherever nature led: more like a man
> Flying from something that he dreads, than one
> Who sought the thing he loved.

And suddenly, as I run, I imagine what it would be like to be responsible for myself—to actually make something of my own life—instead of being obedient to a book or a wife or a lover or a child or even an ideal. And as I strain to grasp this idea, I run on across the strand towards the disappearing sun and back to my family, the people I am hurting most.

And now, as I write this, I wonder: why can't I get it right, that balance, that golden mean that allows us to make our way between equanimity, pain and imagination? Why?

I wonder.

Douglas Bell is a Toronto-born journalist, critic and broadcaster who has worked for *The Globe and Mail*, *Saturday Night*, *Shift*, *Toronto Life*, *The Irish Times* and CBC radio and television. He was hit by a truck on June 10, 1974.

PERMISSIONS

Every effort has been made to contact copyright holders; in the event of an inadvertent omission or error please notify the publisher.

Bishop, Elizabeth. *The Complete Poems: 1927-1979*. Copyright © 1979, 1983 by Alice Helen Methfessel. Copyright © 1933, 1935, 1936, 1937, 1938, 1939, 1940, 1941, 1944, 1945, 1946, 1947, 1948, 1949, 1951, 1952, 1955, 1956, 1957, 1958, 1959, 1960, 1961, 1962, 1963, 1964, 1965, 1966, 1967, 1968, 1969, 1971, 1972, 1973, 1974, 1975, 1976, 1979 by Elizabeth Bishop. Renewal copyright © 1967, 1968, 1971, 1973, 1974, 1975, 1976, 1979 by Elizabeth Bishop. Renewal copyright © 1980 by Alice Helen Methfessel. Published in softcover by Farrar, Straus and Giroux in 1999.

Broyard, Anatole. *Intoxicated by My Illness*. Copyright © 1992 by the Estate of Anatole Broyard. Published in softcover by Ballantine Books in 1993. Reprinted by permission of Random House Inc.

Camus, Albert, as quoted in *Albert Camus: A Life* by Olivier Todd. Copyright © 1997 by Alfred A. Knopf Inc., and copyright © 1996, in different form, by Éditions Gallimard and

Olivier Todd. Published in softcover by Carroll & Graf Publishers, Inc. in 2000.

Cheever, John. *The Journals of John Cheever*. Copyright © 1990, 1991 by Mary Cheever, Susan Cheever, Benjamin Cheever and Federico Cheever. Published in hardcover by Alfred A. Knopf Inc. in 1991. Reprinted by permission of Random House Inc.

Cheever, John. *The Stories of John Cheever*. Copyright © 1946, 1947, 1948, 1949, 1950, 1951, 1952, 1953, 1954, 1955, 1956, 1957, 1958, 1959, 1960, 1961, 1962, 1963, 1964, 1965, 1966, 1967, 1968, 1970, 1972, 1978 by John Cheever. Copyright renewed 1977, 1978 by John Cheever. Published in softcover by Ballantine Books in 1980. Reprinted by permission of Random House Inc.

Kerouac, Jack. *On the Road*. Copyright © 1955, 1957 by Jack Kerouac. Published in softcover by The Viking Press in 1959.

Nuland, Sherman. *How We Die: Reflections on Life's Final Chapter*. Copyright © 1993 by Sherman B. Nuland. Published in softcover by Vintage Books in 1995. Reprinted by permission of Random House Inc.

Rayner, Richard. *The Blue Suit*. Copyright © 1995 by Richard Rayner. Published in softcover by Houghton Mifflin Company in 1995.

Wiesel, Elie. *From the Kingdom of Memory*. Copyright © 1990 by Elirion Associates, Inc. Published in hardcover by Summit Books in 1990.